The Mindful Caregiver

The Mindful Caregiver

Finding Ease in the Caregiving Journey

Nancy L. Kriseman

ROWMAN & LITTLEFIELD
Lanham • Boulder • New York • Toronto • Plymouth, UK

Published by Rowman & Littlefield
4501 Forbes Boulevard, Suite 200, Lanham, Maryland 20706
www.rowman.com

10 Thornbury Road, Plymouth PL6 7PP, United Kingdom

British Library Cataloguing in Publication Information Available

Library of Congress Cataloging-in-Publication Data

The hardback edition of this book was previously catalogued by the Library of Congress as follows:

Kriseman, Nancy L., author.
The mindful caregiver : finding ease in the caregiving journey / by Nancy L. Kriseman.
p. cm.
Includes bibliographical references and index.
[DNLM: 1. Caregivers--psychology. 2. Chronic Disease--rehabilitation. 3. Empathy. 4. Self-Care--methods. 5. Self Care--psychology. WY 200]
RT120.F34 2014
610.73'6--dc23
2013038281

ISBN: 978-1-4422-2354-7 (cloth : alk. paper)
ISBN: 978-1-4422-4869-4 (pbk. : alk. paper)
ISBN: 978-1-4422-2355-4 (electronic)

Printed in the United States of America

To caregivers everywhere, may you find ease in your journey

Contents

Foreword

As you start this book, dear reader, you are entrusting yourself to an experienced and compassionate health professional. Nancy Kriseman has crafted a very practical and heartfelt guide for all of those caregivers who may have wondered at one time or another how they were going to get through the enormous challenges and complexities of caring for a loved one.

As a geriatric social worker with over thirty years of clinical experience and as a caregiver for her mother who had Alzheimer's for seventeen years, Nancy is in a unique position to offer her wisdom on the subject of self-care for the caregiver. As I know from my own experience with my husband who had Alzheimer's, I lived the questions that this book answers. How does one find meaning in what Nancy calls "the tumultuous waters of caregiving?" Where are my sources of support? What can I do when I'm feeling overwhelmed by sadness, resentment, anger, or loss?

Chapter by chapter, *The Mindful Caregiver* sets out to answer these questions in a well-organized, clearly written way. Nancy's book emphasizes two primary approaches to help transform the challenges of caregiving: first, to adopt a practice of mindfulness by being fully present with oneself and one's loved one, and second, to honor what she calls "the spirit-side" of caregiving.

Although mindfulness may be a familiar word to many people, to actually practice mindfulness as a caregiver is an undertaking of immense value; it deepens one's compassion, patience, and kindness—all indispensable qualities for this work. For indeed, it's hard work to be a caregiver! Nancy explains in detail how mindfulness can help you to be more self-aware, gentle, and compassionate with yourself, and bring true presence to your loved one. In addition to helpful self-care exercises, she addresses a wide variety of subjects such as expectations, decision making, advocacy, resources, and perhaps most important of all, how to deepen the relationship with your care recipient.

The Mindful Caregiver is a treasury of gifts for you, the caregiver.

In addition to all of the book's creative ideas, I love that Nancy was adventurous enough to break out of assumed roles about how one "should" provide caregiving. She gives a compelling example of how she was present to her mother during the last bed-ridden stages of illness, a story I'll leave for you to discover.

Nancy's commitment to the field of caregiving is inspiring. Her book will provide guidance, encouragement, and inspiration for how to find ease in the caregiving journey. By emphasizing both mindfulness and the spiritual dimension, she shows how to reap the gifts of caregiving, honor the precious moments, and ennoble the challenges. Her book will help caregivers find the courage to follow their unique paths through what can be both the most challenging yet heartwarming experience of a lifetime.

Olivia Ames Hoblitzelle, *Ten Thousand Joys & Ten Thousand Sorrows: A Couple's Journey through Alzheimer's*
Cambridge, Massachusetts
July 2013

Preface

Travelers there is no path; paths are made by walking.
— Antonio Machado, nineteenth-century Spanish poet

MINDFULNESS AND THE "MINDFUL CAREGIVER"

I am a geriatric social worker who has counseled and supported caregivers and their family members, friends, and others who have sought care. I also am the daughter of a mother who lived with Alzheimer's disease for seventeen years. In my thirty-plus years of clinical practice, I have worked with many caregivers who have been challenged by many different chronic diseases. Time after time, they shared with me how exhausted and frustrated they felt caring for their family member, loved one, or, as we call it in the field, "care recipient." Some even expressed anger and resentment because they had to place their lives on hold.

When I asked how they were taking care of themselves, I would repeatedly hear: "I am having a hard enough time providing care. How can I even think about taking care of myself?" Knowing that so many caregivers felt helpless and hopeless, I became motivated to help my clients travel the caregiver path in a more balanced and less agonizing way.

About midway through my career, my seventy-one-year-old mother was diagnosed with Alzheimer's disease. As I began the caregiving journey with my own mother, I realized how important it was to take care of myself while also caring for her. I asked myself: What did I expect of myself? How would I take care of myself? What did my family expect of me? How would I stay connected to my mother when her disease became worse? How would this experience affect my ability to help others?

I became even more motivated to help myself and my clients find balance and navigate this new, unfamiliar territory with a little more ease. It was in that spirit that I developed the notion of being a "mindful caregiver." Being *mindful* meant traveling the caregiver path with intentionality. To accomplish this, I needed to check in with myself on a regular basis to make sure I was attending to my physical, emotional, and spiritual health.

As I reflect back, I realize that using a mindful approach to caring for my mother incorporated the concepts of what is now called *mindfulness*. Today, mindfulness is a well-researched approach to taking care of oneself in a more balanced and healthy way. Throughout this book, I provide many ideas, strategies, and case examples of how to be a mindful caregiver.

How Mindfulness Can Help You

> There is no right or wrong way to provide care. However, a mindfulness approach can help ease the way.

This book provides caregivers with a different lens through which to view caregiving—the lens of mindfulness. Mindfulness can help bring self-awareness into focus. It reminds you that *you matter!* It nudges you to be kind and gentle, nonjudgmental, and compassionate with yourself. It can help you prioritize, set limits, stay true to yourself, and ultimately feel more at ease during the caregiving journey.

When you approach caregiving more *mindfully* you can:

- Feel more at ease as you travel down the caregiver path.
- View each stressful situation as an opportunity to learn how to *pause, take a step back,* and then *proceed with caution*—instead of just jumping right in.
- Learn a wider range of caregiving practices. All kinds of ideas, options, and opportunities await you!
- Realize that there is no longer a right or wrong way to provide care, only a more mindful way.

A Daughter's View of Being a Mindful Caregiver

I knew the journey with my mother would be difficult and depressing at times. Now I had the opportunity to be "up close" to this disease. I realized my challenges would be similar to those faced by my clients. So I took on this new role with determination to stay connected to myself, my mother, and my clients. I also hoped to gain insights on how to best help all of us.

My first commitment to being a *mindful caregiver* was paying close attention to how *I was feeling.* I knew that I had to nurture myself throughout my caregiving journey with my mom. I did my best to keep my spirit as positive as possible under the circumstances. I was committed to finding joy, humor, and love so that I could appreciate the true blessings that caring for someone can bring forth. Yet I also knew I had to embrace the more difficult aspects of caregiving. I faced feelings of sadness, anger, and loss. And I learned the importance of setting limits to make sure I didn't lose myself and my life to my mother's illness. Finding balance meant allowing all of the above to shine through.

Additionally, I realized that my mother's disease could wreak havoc on her spirit. I thought about all the various ways to connect to my mother's spirit, and being a mindful caregiver inspired me to reach deep into my heart and soul. I learned to be silly, to sing, and to laugh with my mother. I realized it didn't matter whether she said the right word or didn't know where she was. I had to be willing to let go of the rigid places in myself. I learned to live more in the moment and be with her in a simpler way, which provided much more enjoyment for both of us. I also learned to more effectively cope with the difficult times, when Mom would become agitated or sad, and at times, even mean. I gave myself permission to feel sad, upset, or just plain tired of dealing with her illness. Validating my feelings helped me let them go more easily. I share my story because it is easy to have high expectations and envision what your caregiving experience should be. Holding onto expectations can set you up for significant stress and burnout. Not acknowledging emotions can add to an already heavy heart. When you are able to shake your high expectations and acknowledge your feelings, you can more easily let go and embrace new ways to "be" with your care recipient. This approach helped keep my spirit alive and allowed me to walk the caregiver path with more ease. Likewise, many caregivers in my practice were helped by this approach.

This book could not have been written without the amazing caregivers I have met. They have bestowed so many blessings on me as I traveled with them through the tumultuous waters of caregiving. It is in their honor that I write this book and share the knowledge they gifted me. I am hopeful that as you read the various chapters, you will walk away with new ideas and ways to approach your role as caregiver.

Namaste,
Nancy L. Kriseman, LCSW

Acknowledgments

It takes a village to support an author. I have been blessed to have been truly supported by a village of amazing people.

My book village, Rowman & Littlefield, made this book possible. I would like to start by saying a special thanks to Suzanne Staszak-Silva, my submissions publisher, who believed in the concept of *The Mindful Caregiver* and shepherded the manuscript into a book. Thank you to Elaine McGarraugh and Kathryn Knigge who were supportive, responsive, and kindhearted.

I am so grateful to all my family, friends, and work colleagues, too many to mention by name. They listened with caring ears and helped keep my spirit positive. And, of course, all the remarkable caregivers I have worked with over the past thirty years. They are true inspirations!

There are two special people that I would like to thank. Kerry Kriseman, my sister-in-law, who didn't hesitate when I told her I needed someone to help edit the beginning chapters of my book. She gave me encouragement that enabled me to move forward. Cynthia Jorgensen, DrPH, my life partner, whose unending love, support, and belief in me helped sustain me through the sometimes arduous task of writing. She was my "editor in chief," offering endless hours of her time and expertise "weeding through my garden" so my "words could bloom." She provided invaluable assistance, organizing my content and ensuring its accuracy, enabling readers to walk away with the best possible information.

My "angel" book colleague was Olivia Hoblitzelle, whose loving and generous spirit offered wisdom and guidance. She nurtured my spirit, especially when I was feeling overwhelmed. She is a true "caring spirit."

Annie Rosetti, my graduate student researcher, whose careful eyes and superb organizational skills helped me research all my references and quotes. She was always willing to look up "one more thing."

Toco Hills Avis G. Williams librarians, Leslie Barber and Elizabeth Isabelle were relentless in doing all they could to find the references I needed.

Bonnie Cooper my dearest friend and social work colleague who was my cheerleader and faithful supporter. She was always there for me no matter when I called her and provided a compassionate ear and precise, prudent suggestions. Mary Erlanger PhD, my wise sage, who pushed me to rethink some of my content. Both were my professional readers, providing instrumental suggestions about content, organization, and clarity.

They read through the unedited versions of my manuscript, which required tireless patience and time.

My family caregiver readers, Sandy Simon and Leigh Tompros, your ideas and suggestions were invaluable, as you were in the caregiving trenches.

Dan Munster and Connie Buffington, both attorneys, despite their busy practices and lives, provided expert legal advice for the book.

I am forever grateful to have been able to write much of my book in the glorious splendor of the Toco Hills Avis G. Williams Library. My cozy corner overlooking the beautiful forest was inspirational! And to the Mercer University pool that was a very calming source of comfort and rejuvenation.

Introduction

How to Become a Mindful Caregiver

> Mindfulness is the aware, balanced acceptance of the present experience. It isn't more complicated than that. It is opening to or receiving the present moment, pleasant or unpleasant, just as it is, without either clinging to it or rejecting it.
> —Sylvia Boorstein, *It's Easier Than You Think,* 101

HOW MINDFULNESS CAN HELP

I wrote this book to help caregivers find ways to take better care of themselves. Many caregivers share that they often feel alone, isolated, and unappreciated. *Mindfulness* can offer renewed hope for finding support and value for your role as a caregiver. Mindfulness requires that you pay attention to how you feel in the present moment and that you do so in a nonjudgmental way. It requires that you slow down and connect to your heart so that you can more fully experience yourself and the life around you. Mindfulness embraces the qualities of compassion, kindness, and patience. It is an approach that everyone can use. It can help slow you down some so you can make the best possible decisions for your care recipient. It also helps bring more balance and ease while navigating the caregiving journey.

Being a mindful caregiver requires paying attention to how caregiving impacts *you.* When you apply mindfulness to caregiving, you are able to:

- Be intentional about the care you provide and the time you spend with your care recipient.
- Be aware of all your emotions and feelings and how they affect you.
- Recognize your relationship to the care recipient for what it is.
- Travel your own unique path, without being critical or judgmental of yourself and your feelings.
- Stay in the present moment with openness and acceptance.
- Recognize that you cannot be responsible for all of the care that your care recipient needs.

Ignoring or denying how caregiving affects you can set you up for burnout and numb-out. Mindfulness brings attention back to you so you don't lose yourself in the caregiving process. It enables you to take positive action. You learn to find ways to take care of yourself as you provide care to your care recipient. In the geriatric field, individuals that require care are called "care recipients," which is the term I use throughout this book. For some of you, the care recipient will be a spouse, partner, or family member. Others may find themselves caring for a friend or loved one. What is hopeful about this practice is that there are many easy ways to incorporate mindfulness practices into your day-to-day caregiving routines.

MINDFULNESS AND THE SPIRIT-SIDE OF CARING

We thrive when we feel intimately connected heart to heart and soul to soul.

—Paula Reeves, *Heart Sense*, 101

An important aspect of mindfulness is recognizing the *spirit-side* of caregiving. It requires awareness of how your emotions impact your spirit and vice versa. Let me explain.

The spirit is the essence of a person. It is a force or energy inside and outside of you. Your spirit helps you stay connected to your heart and what really matters to you.

When you feel spirited, you often feel uplifted, happy, at ease, joyful, and connected. When you feel *dispirited*, you can become depressed, unengaged, unmotivated, tired, easily angered, inpatient, and unhappy. Thus, your spirit has a great impact on your emotions. Integrating mindfulness into the caregiving experience makes tending to your spirit and whole well-being a priority. You learn to let go of the aspects of caregiving that deplete your spirit and cause emotional pain and suffering.

Consider the following question: How often do you feel guilty that you are not doing enough? From my experience, many caregivers become stressed out, thinking they need to be doing more. They tend to get caught in an unrealistic pattern of continuing to doing more for the care recipient until they wear themselves down. However, when your spirit is strong, you are able to set realistic expectations so you don't wear yourself out. You acknowledge your guilt and then let it go so that it doesn't overtake you. When your spirit is strong, you are able to be more resilient. Utilizing a mindfulness approach encourages you to make sure you nurture the spirit-side of yourself. In doing so, you can more effectively handle the many challenges you face. Nurturing your spirit-side helps fortify you.

The spirit-side of caregiving can be beneficial to the care recipient as well. Finding ways to connect to your care recipient's spirit can ease him or her. No matter how ill, your care recipient's spirit tunes into your energy and reacts to your emotions, whether you are angry, anxious, joyful, or calm. Thus when you are more at ease, often your care recipient will be more at ease. When you are both comfortable, your experience together can take on new meaning and purpose. When you connect to each other's spirits, the relationship between you and the care recipient can deepen.

To best help you understand how mindfulness and the spirit-side of caregiving can impact your experience, let me present several case examples. You will be introduced to some self-care techniques that are explained in later chapters. The first case example is my own experience with my mother. The others are of a son, a spouse, and a care recipient. All the case examples in this book are real situations. I have changed the names and some of the personal information to ensure privacy. It is my hope that these examples will encourage you to read on and learn how these approaches can be helpful to you.

EXAMPLES OF THE IMPACT OF MINDFULNESS AND THE SPIRIT-SIDE OF CARING

My Own Experience as a Daughter

When my mother was first diagnosed with Alzheimer's disease (AD), my intuition said this strong, feisty woman would live with this disease a long time. How right I was! She lived with Alzheimer's for seventeen years. I knew in my heart that I had to keep my spirit alive if I was to be of any support to her. I made a commitment to stay mindful throughout my journey with my mom. I would make the time, no matter how life tried to get in my way, to tend to my spirit! *I kept it simple.*

- I remembered to take deep breaths, which helped calm and center me.
- I made time for relaxation. Even ten minutes can help. I listened to soothing music, found a quiet place in my house to just sit, spent time outdoors soaking in the beauty of nature, or took a long, hot bath instead of a shower.
- I stayed connected to the friends and family who nourished me, and I avoided those who depleted me.
- I made time for my two most joyful hobbies, gardening and photography.
- I honored my weekly date with my then-two-year-old nephew, Adam.
- I continued to work out, which always gave me pleasure and relieved much stress.
- I sought out different religious and spiritual practices that helped keep me centered and, quite frankly, sane.

All the ways I took care of myself may not be helpful to you. You have to find your own path. However, my goal in this book is to provide a variety of ways that can help you navigate the caregiving journey. In subsequent chapters, I explain these in more depth.

While taking care of myself and connecting to my spirit, I wanted to find a way to connect to my mother's spirit as well. As her AD became more severe, she reached a point in which she was more confused, less alert, and less comfortable sitting in her wheelchair. In this phase of her illness, I would often find her in bed. It was very difficult to connect and interact with her. It felt uncomfortable to see her lying in bed while I sat up and looked down at her. My heart ached for us both. I missed our more active times and all the ways we had connected to one another in the past. After several agonizing visits, I realized I needed to find a new way for both our spirits to connect.

First, I had to honor my sad feelings about how the way we had related to each other had changed. Then I became determined to find new ways to enjoy being with each other. One way was to just get in bed with her. I can only imagine what many caregivers may think as they read this. A fifty-year-old daughter lying in bed with her mother, how unusual is that? For me, however, it was a special experience that I will always cherish. While lying in bed with Mom, we hummed songs, held hands, and learned to "just be" with one another. It helped make my visit much more enjoyable, and I truly believe she enjoyed herself as well. She was calm and peaceful during those times. I am convinced that taking care of my own spirit helped me stay more connected to my mother. I will be eternally grateful for the ways it transformed our journey.

This experience, however, helped me recognize that whenever possible I would help caregivers find new ways of communicating and connecting. I believed that caregivers could have less stressful and more meaningful experiences.

Michael: A Son's Experience

I worked with Michael, whose father had Alzheimer's disease. He and his father had always been quite close. Now, however, Michael shared that he was having a very difficult time connecting to his father, who had a limited attention span and short-term memory. His father would ask the same questions or repeat the same story over and over. Michael dreaded his visits because he didn't feel as if they had much of a reciprocal relationship anymore.

I asked him what sorts of activities they had enjoyed together over the years and if they had any shared interests. He mentioned that they used to enjoy woodworking projects and going to car shows, but his father was no longer able to enjoy those activities. Thinking about their past interests, I suggested that they look through car magazines together, make a car collage of their favorite cars, or maybe watch auto races together on television.

Michael became a mindful caregiver, recognizing the importance of planning his visits with his father in order to make the time they spent together more meaningful and enjoyable. Michael mentioned that his visits had become much more pleasant.

Mandy: A Spouse's Experience

Mandy contacted me regarding her husband, Ben. Her husband of thirty years had Parkinson's and Alzheimer's disease. He was fifteen years older than she and, although they had no children, he had a son by his first marriage. The son was not very involved and lived out of town. She reluctantly decided to have Ben evaluated to determine if she should care for him at home or would need to move him into a nursing home.

Mandy had cared for Ben by herself for a number of years, but over time it was becoming increasingly more difficult. She gradually hired more and more caregivers to help. She mentioned missing her privacy and said her home felt like a nursing home with all the round-the-clock care. Yet, at the same time, she liked the closeness and ability to spend time with Ben. She shared that the thought of moving him to a nursing home weighed heavily on her heart. For more than a year, her brother had been telling her that she needed to move her husband into a nursing home. He was particularly worried about her health and quality of life. Most spousal caregivers rarely consider their own health. This was the case with Mandy. It is not unusual for spousal caregivers to resist seeking help or making changes.

I asked Mandy if she might consider a different way to think about her situation. Would she be willing to be a mindful caregiver? I explained what was meant by being mindful. Her first order of business was to check in with herself about how *she* was doing. Being a mindful caregiver meant tending to herself as well as her husband. She agreed to give this approach a try.

Mandy had several sessions in which we created the sacred space for her to "be" with her feelings. I reminded her that being mindful requires that she slow down in order to connect to her heart. As she shared her feelings, I emphasized that honoring all emotions helps honor their relationship. In her situation, her relationship was one both she and her husband had treasured. She affirmed how much they had loved, respected, and appreciated each other throughout their marriage. Although she knew her husband now needed to be in a nursing home, she worried about how he would manage emotionally without her. She knew he had to be in a place where he could receive the best care. Through many tears, she was able to connect to her heart. She realized that she would be more at ease knowing her husband would receive the constant medical care that could not be provided at home. She also admitted rather meekly that she would love to have her house back again.

Once her decision was made, I helped Mandy develop a thoughtful transition plan for Ben. The plan involved providing ways to best ease her and her husband as they both adjusted to the nursing home. The plan also included providing helpful information to the staff. In addition, I encouraged her to create a warm and comfortable environment in his room by bringing in some of his favorite furniture, pictures, and other items that they both enjoyed. She brought some fragrant incense to make the room more inviting. Lastly, we discussed different ways to make her visits as meaningful as possible for both of them. This was particularly important, because as her husband declined, she would need to plan for different ways to visit and be with him. (Chapter 5 focuses on how to visit and communicate with your care recipient.)

In our time together, Mandy shared how helpful it was to approach caring for her husband in a more mindful, spirit-focused way. Being an amazingly loving spouse, she was willing to be open to finding new ways to be in his life. She sang with him, read him funny short stories, and brought in music that they both enjoyed and often danced to. As time went on, Ben declined more. He was placed on hospice care. Although I knew this would be difficult and very sad, I was also encouraged that she would find new ways for them to stay connected. She brought in soothing music, and would lower the lights, light lavender candles, and just lie in bed with him or sit next to him and hold his hand. Mandy shared how special the last few weeks were with her husband. While she felt extremely sad, she mentioned how spending time in that way seemed to create even more closeness between the two of them. I shared a Native American quote, which she found much comfort in. I hope this quote will comfort you too: "The soul would have no rainbow if the eyes had no tears."[1]

Rebecca: A Caregiver and Care Recipient's Experience

Early in my career, ninety-one-year-old Rebecca taught me about the importance of the spirit and being mindful of how the spirit helps keep you connected to others. She was a volunteer at the nursing home where my mother lived. Every day, Rebecca walked from her independent apartment building to the attached nursing home to help feed the elders who could not feed themselves. One night, as I visited my mother, I found Rebecca sitting with my mother helping cut her food and joking with her. I watched the two interact and observed the beautiful way their spirits connected with one another. Rebecca seemed unfazed by Mom's dementia. I was very touched by Rebecca's kind heart, warm smile, and positive energy. From that point on, for the next ten years, Rebecca and I became dear friends. I learned a lot about this wonderfully spirited, elder woman. She had been in the Army and served as a volunteer nurse. Rebecca fought her way through many illnesses and was widowed three times. She never had children but won the heart of all her nieces and nephews, who would do anything for her. She survived the death of her beloved niece, who was like a daughter to her. She took care of several of her ailing sisters until their deaths. And later in her life, she volunteered for the Atlanta Symphony because of her love for music.

Even after Rebecca could no longer drive due to poor eyesight and difficulty walking, the Atlanta Symphony administrator sent a taxi to pick up this special volunteer. I was dazzled by Rebecca's positive spirit and ability to keep it so alive. One day I found the nerve to ask her what kept her spirit going. She laughed, "I surround myself with people and things that nurture my spirit and keep me going. You have to do the things that give you joy and be around people that you love and that love you."

It was in that moment that I realized how vital connections of the spirit are. Rebecca serves as a reminder of how the spirit-side of caring facilitates staying connected to oneself, to others, and to the world around us. Even now, Rebecca's spirit is still felt by those who loved her.

I hope these examples have inspired you to consider how mindfulness and the spirit-side of caregiving can open new pathways for you and your care recipient.

Remember the message throughout this book: *You matter!*

NOTES

1. Guy Zona, *The Soul Would Have No Rainbow If the Eyes Had No Tears* (New York: Simon & Schuster, 1994).

ONE

Understanding the Caregiver Role

The Mindful Caregiver

Caregiving will never be one-size-fits-all.

When my mother was diagnosed with Alzheimer's disease, it seemed obvious that as a geriatric social worker I would be the best person to serve as my mother's power of attorney for health care. I had more than fifteen years of experience at the time, and my brother, although living closer to my mother, agreed that as "the geriatric professional," I would be more suited to help and advocate for her. I helped place our mother in an assisted living community in Florida, although my brother and I agreed that when our mother required nursing home care, we would move her to Atlanta. Mother adjusted well to the assisted living community and lived there for almost two years. Then she had a stroke and ended up in the hospital. Once she was stable, we made arrangements to move her to Atlanta, and she moved into the nursing home where I had worked as a social worker.

Once in Atlanta, I naively believed that my professional experience (and location) would make my role as my mother's advocate and health-care manager easy. While my geriatric social work training was helpful, I was not as prepared for the emotional aspects of this role. Spending much time with her and making decisions about her care quickly made me realize how easily my emotions could get in my way. In the beginning, I must admit, my emotions got the best of me and I found it difficult to make decisions. At times I felt guilty that I couldn't take care of her on my own and sad that she had to be in a nursing home. I became cognizant of how much easier it was to hide behind the professional hat, as I could push my emotional feelings aside and focus on "what needed to be done." Yet, I also knew that as her disease worsened over time, it would be more difficult to push my emotional feelings aside. I suspected that that my emotions and mother's situation could greatly impact my spirit as well. I began to realize it would be critical for me to find ways to nourish my spirit.

As I journeyed down the path of caregiver-advocate, I realized what mattered most was figuring out how to preserve my spirit. For me, that meant maintaining our mother–daughter relationship. As long as I could, I wanted to find ways to still feel my mother was my mother, and I, her daughter. Even toward the end of her disease, I treated her as my mother and continued to share aspects about my life. While many outside observers may think otherwise, in my heart, I believe our hearts and spirit remained connected. As a caregiver, your emotions can easily get in the way of providing care and making decisions. For instance, when you are feeling depressed, angry, frustrated, or guilty, the emotional charge may make it difficult to make decisions or to make the best ones. It is not unusual for your spirit to be impacted as well. When you feel a lack of spirit, your negative emotions quickly rise to the top. As a result, your caregiving journey can leave you feeling exhausted and sad. In contrast, when your spirit feels alive, you often feel uplifted, more positive, and more at ease. You have more energy to cope. Being mindful of your emotions and spirit is critical to lessening your stress and helping you feel more empowered.

This chapter discusses what the caregiver role can encompass. When caregivers become more aware of the different aspects of their roles, they have increased opportunities to take better care of themselves.

DEFINING YOUR CAREGIVER ROLE AS A MINDFUL CAREGIVER

I would venture to guess that most caregivers probably didn't think too much about what it means to be a caregiver until they found themselves in this role. Most caregivers haven't been trained nor have they had many role models. I have found that many people learn caregiving from the seat of their pants without much planning or guidance. There are many different aspects and approaches to caregiving, and unfortunately, a "one-size-fits-all" method does not exist.

In my thirty-plus years practicing, I have helped caregivers define their roles and recognize that each journey is unique. I have tried to empower them and to educate them about what this new role entails. With an understanding of what to realistically expect and manage, I believe that caregivers have a greater likelihood of success, and perhaps most importantly, a greater likelihood of managing their stress.

For starters, it is an important point to keep in mind how you entered into this role. Many caregivers have been thrust into this role out of pure necessity or obligation. Some may feel ambivalent, while others may feel resentment or anger. There will those adults who may choose not to provide care but instead to hire someone to act on their behalf. Others will be those who will decide to opt out completely. There are even people who may have been abused or neglected by the care recipient for whom they now have to provide care. And some caregivers entered into this role truly out of love.

Whichever of the above describes you, keep in mind that the caregiver role can be influenced by a number of different factors:

- How you entered into this role
- Your past and present relationship with the person
- Your personality and the personality of the care recipient
- Your current life situation
- The support or lack of support available to you
- Your financial resources
- Your own health and the health of the person you are caring for

These are some of the factors that influence the caregiver role. Being mindful of the above can help you define a role that is both realistic and congruent with your desires. Please keep in mind, however, that each caregiver will have to make her own unique path in this journey.

HOW CARING FOR AN OLDER ADULT IS DIFFERENT

As you begin your role as caregiver, it's important to point out that caring for older adults is very different than caring for children. When I shared the challenges of caring for my mother, many of my friends seemed to believe that caring for adults was similar to caring for children. The differences couldn't be more profound. Children, in most circumstances, are healthy and grow and mature, whereas elders are on the opposite path. Adults look forward to watching their children grow competent and independent. In contrast, older adults grow frail and more dependent. Watching an elder lose competency is not something to look forward to. And what I find disturbing is that we tend to label caring for older adults as a "drain" or "burden." In contrast, the words "burden" or "drain" rarely come up when we talk about caring for children.

My experiences with my mother and the caregivers with whom I have worked have helped me recognize that one of the most gut-wrenching aspects of caring for an older adult is coping with their loss of capacity. This can be very hard to acknowledge, let alone accept. I will never forget the time I shared with a dear friend of mine how upset I was when my mother became incontinent. I felt sad and upset about my mother no longer being able to use the toilet on her own. Expecting compassion, she quickly retorted back, "Nancy, that's really no big deal. Why don't you just try to think of her situation like you would of a child?" She truly thought there was no difference. I knew she meant well, but I was angry. How dare she think these situations were similar? I felt that she didn't understand how painful and sad it is when an adult, especially your parent, loses the capacity to care for herself. It was in that moment I knew that it would be important to point out these differences to the caregivers with whom I worked. Helping caregivers acknowledge their feelings about what it felt like to care for an adult would be critical to their being able to find more ease.

I am also reminded of another stark example of these differences. To this day, I can still remember the irony I felt thinking about the care needs of my mother and my niece, Jordan. Jordan was fifteen months old, and we were all excited and proud that she had recently taken her first steps. Yet, in the same time period, my mother lost her ability to walk. My mother, who had walked several miles every day of her life, was now not even able to take one step on her own. As elated as I was about my niece's new developmental milestones, I was equally deflated and distressed by the developmental losses my mother was experiencing. My niece was gaining new skills and my mother was losing skills along with her independence. Having to acknowledge my mother's losses definitely challenged my ability to keep my spirit positive and calm. I hope my lessons will help other caregivers find a way to become as resilient.

CAREGIVER ROLE DIFFERENCES

As differences exist between caring for a younger versus older person, likewise there are differences between adult children caregivers and spousal caregivers. The relationships and feelings that adult children and spouses experience when caring for recipient are clearly very different. It's important to be aware of the unique role distinctions. I have therefore created two separate sections, one for spousal caregivers and one for adult children caregivers.

Spouse/Partner Caregivers

> "My husband's disease has created a man I don't even recognize. I love my husband, but I am not sure how long I can continue to care for him at home. When I share my concerns, my children don't seem to understand."
>
> —Words from a loving spouse

In my practice, I have repeatedly seen that spouses from the Traditionalist generation, those born before 1945, strongly hold to the marriage vows of "In sickness and in health, until death do us part." Many are willing to sacrifice their own health in order to honor those wedding vows. They expect that spouses *should* take care of each other and *tough it out*. There-fore, it's no surprise that spouses of this generation adamantly believe they have to remain steadfast and by their spouse's side throughout the entire illness.

As a husband or wife, there are many ways to support and care for your spouse that won't jeopardize your own life and health. First, let's examine the most common challenges you may confront along your jour-ney and learn some strategies on how to cope with some of them.

Changes in Your Physical Well-Being and Resilience

It is a well-known fact that as you age, your physical energy and stamina often decrease. You tend to be less resilient, and it can take more time to recover from stress or illness. In addition, you may have your own physical issues, which can greatly influence your ability to provide care to your ill spouse. Managing an ill or frail spouse's activities of daily living, such as bathing your spouse or lifting her out of a chair or off the toilet, can place you in physical danger. I have witnessed too many care-giving spouses, particularly those who are older, completely ignore ma-jor warning signs about their own health and become ill themselves. It is well documented that caregivers who don't take care of themselves are much more prone to becoming ill.[1] And even more tragically, I have known a few caregivers who died while trying to take care of their spouse. I share this not to scare you but to remind you of the conse-quences if you don't take care of yourself.

Spousal caregivers have to be particularly mindful of how much care they can *realistically* provide while also considering their own physical resources. A mindful caregiver recognizes that *you can't do everything* for your care recipient. You have to allow others to help out. And I would like to offer you something to consider. Allowing others to help provides your spouse with the opportunity to interact with other loving people. You spouse can benefit from the social interaction with others. Realizing you are not the only one who can provide loving care may be uncomfort-able at first. As author Marty Richards describes in her book *Caresharing*, "sharing the care" can open many doors for both you and your spouse.[2]

Placement Considerations—Moving Your Spouse

There are so many issues to consider, it is no wonder many spousal caregivers put this issue off as long as possible.

Deciding whether to move your spouse to a care facility is an issue that unfortunately is all too common and one that gives spousal caregiv-ers considerable angst. Moving your spouse can evoke strong feelings, which can make this decision especially difficult. In my experience, the majority of well spouses don't want to move into a care facility with their ill spouse, as it means giving up their home, community, and independence. And if the well spouse and ill spouse have different care needs, it is not always easy to find a facility that can accommodate the two different situations. Furthermore, if you find a community that can, it often means having to pay two rental fees—one for each living situation.

Very often, caregivers hold fear deep in their hearts when thinking about placing their spouse. In fact, fear and guilt are often the biggest barriers when trying to make a decision about moving a spouse. In my practice, I have found that most caregivers experience one or the other, and sometimes both. In addition, a common belief is that your spouse will decline more quickly if moved into an assisted living or nursing home. It's no wonder that so many caregivers are terrified. While it is possible that your spouse could decline, this generally is not the case if you find a suitable place for your care recipient. But it does take careful research and proactive planning. You have to advocate for your spouse and ensure that a good transition plan is in place. These topics are discussed in depth in chapter 7, "Being a Partner and Advocate in Care." When families take these steps, the move can be much less traumatic.

Now let's take a look at guilt and how it factors into making this decision. Unfortunately, many spousal caregivers are their own worst enemies when it comes to harboring guilt. What I mean by this is that you place unrealistic expectations on yourselves. You believe you have to care for your spouse at home and that you should be able to do so, no matter how ill he becomes. As a result, guilt arises for a number of reasons. You may feel as if you have failed as a caregiver if you aren't able to keep your spouse at home. Or you see other caregivers who are able to keep their spouse at home and you wonder what is wrong with you. Perhaps you feel pressure from family members or friends to keep your spouse at home. Or lastly, you may have unresolved feelings about your spouse that "guilt trip" you into thinking you should care for your spouse at home. Being able to manage your guilt and recognize how it can become a barrier to making decisions takes courage. And it can take *even more courage* to admit when you can no longer care for your ill spouse at home.

It is critical to be mindful of how you *give life* to your guilt. When you give life to your guilt, you can feel anxious, depressed, and stressed. Those feelings can interfere with making a realistic decision. When caregivers use a mindfulness approach, they can learn new ways to cope. Mindfulness requires that you acknowledge your guilt, but you don't judge it. You just allow yourself to be with the feelings. For example, you may want to take some deep breaths to calm yourself down. You accept the guilt and begin to realize it doesn't have to overtake you. You breathe in, acknowledge the guilt, and then let it go. Guilt will "come to visit" every so often. However, mindful caregivers learn to recognize its presence and then compassionately release it, so they can do what is best for themselves and their care recipient.

After becoming aware of how fear and guilt can get in the way of making good decisions, the next step is gathering as much support around you as possible. Having someone else help you decide to place your spouse in a facility can relieve some of the guilt and stress that you may feel. If you have family, reach out to them. If you don't, or aren't able to talk with family members, perhaps you can engage your care recipient's doctor. In difficult situations, such as complex cases in which there is significant family conflict or resistance, I recommend that you consider joining a support group or hiring a professional. Sometimes being with others who are wrestling with similar issues can be comforting, informative, and empowering. Professionals can be helpful as they can provide objectivity.

Placement Considerations—Deciding to Not Move Your Spouse

There will be some spousal caregivers who determine that it is best to not move their spouse. Some spousal caregivers will try to keep their spouse at home, becoming the primary caregiver. Other spousal caregivers may consider hiring in some help. Keeping your spouse at home can be successfully accomplished with careful planning. (Chapter 6 has a section on what you need to think about if keeping your care recipient at home.) You have to be mindful of how trying to take care of your spouse can have adverse effects on *your* health and well-being. It will be critical that you find ways to share the care with others so you have some replenishing time.

In order to provide adequate care, you may need to hire in-home caregivers, if you can afford it. (Chapter 6 has a section on Home Care.) Or you will need to find creative ways to find help. Let's look at in-home paid caregiver support first. Having in-home caregivers requires a certain amount of management, especially if you hire a person on your own. It will be important for you to determine exactly what you would like the in-home caregiver to do for you and your spouse. You need to be clear in your goals and your needs. Do you know what you will do if the caregiver gets sick, stuck in traffic, or just doesn't show up? Even if you use a home care service, you will have to keep up with who is coming, when they are coming, what each person will be doing, and what supplies they may need. And even with outside caregiver support, you are living with your spouse day in and day out. As a side note, a number of spousal caregivers have shared that having outside caregivers in their home was the most difficult aspect of providing care for their spouse. They felt as if they had no privacy. Whenever possible, it will be important to have some alone time in your house without the caregiver and your spouse. Plan times where the caregiver takes your spouse out of the house for a few hours. Many spouses have shared how helpful it was to have time to just be in their own house, perhaps to quietly read a book or take a bath, with no one else around. If you can't afford paid help, explore whether there are volunteer programs that provide trained visitors who can stay with your care recipient for an hour or two. These programs, when available, are often offered by your local Office on Aging, as well as by some churches and other faith groups. In addition, find out if there might be university students who would be willing to volunteer their time.

Whether you end up moving your spouse or keeping her at home, each situation requires careful consideration. A decision to move your spouse or keep her at home has to be in the best interests of both you and your care recipient.

Relationship Changes

In most caregiving situations, your relationship with your spouse will change. Learning to live with a spouse who has a chronic disease or disability requires being willing to make adjustments that are often unfamiliar and awkward at first. Accommodating to this new phase of your life as a couple is a process that will take some time. In fact, psychologist Joseph Nowinski, coauthor of *Saying Goodbye: How Families Can Find Renewal through Loss*, refers to this life stage as "the new grief" and states that "new grief" has resulted from modern medicine's ability to arrest or slow down terminal illness, thus keeping people alive for years on end.[3] And it can keep caregivers on an emotional roller-coaster. You have to adjust to a host of changes that can cause grief-like symptoms, such as sadness, anger, impatience, and at times even despair. These changes require that you shift role responsibilities and adjust to new ways of communicating and being intimate with one another. I recall a spousal caregiver who shared that she struggled with letting go of the "we" part of their relationship. Even though her husband was in a nursing home, she would still talk to friends, family, or professionals using the vernacular "we." Thinking about herself as more of an "I" filled her with great sadness. I suggested that she slowly begin to transition to "I" and do so when it felt least upsetting.

One of the major changes that spousal caregivers face, which can be the most uncomfortable and upsetting, is how to cope with intimacy. Intimacy is a very personal and private matter for couples. In my work with spousal caregivers, many have shared how awkward they feel discussing this topic with their friends, family, and even their physician. Being emotionally and physically close is a human desire and a lifelong need. Intimacy in couples is often what defines the relationship as sacred and special. In most circumstances, sexual contact and frequency will change when your spouse becomes ill. Many spouses who had positive loving relationships mention how much they miss the physical intimacy they used to have with their spouse. I do encourage spouses to continue to touch, hug, and lie in bed together, as they can still derive pleasure from being with one another. In addition to the physical closeness, spouses also mention missing the sharing of intimate thoughts and feelings with one another. They yearn for the give and take of their relationship, and the sharing of holidays, birthdays, and other celebrations. Ultimately, you will need to acknowledge these losses and the sadness associated with them. You have to give yourself permission to grieve these losses.

While you may not be able to replace the special intimacy of a spouse, you may be able to find and experience different kinds of intimacy. Make sure you stay connected to people whom you love and who love you. Let your friends and family know when you would like a hug. Consider cuddling with a grandchild or a loving pet. You might also consider nurturing your body by getting massages, taking baths, or spending time in nature. In some situations, some spouses may find a lover who can replace the sexual intimacy that they miss. Whether you discuss this with your ill spouse depends on a number of factors—for example, if your spouse has significant cognitive impairment or the nature of your relationship is not one to encourage such a discussion. Only you can determine what feels right and comfortable for your situation. This issue can certainly bring up some guilt feelings. It may be helpful for you to talk with either a counselor or spiritual professional. These are different ways to find physical intimacy and they are unique for each caregiver. Emotional and social intimacy can be somewhat replaced by time with friends and family, finding hobbies, or perhaps volunteering for a special cause. Intimacy of all types helps to stoke your spirit and keeps you connected to the life around and within you. Navigating through your role as a spousal caregiver can bring new ways of connecting that can be enjoyable and life altering.

Adult Children Caregivers

"In the face of an elder's increasingly complex and protracted caregiving needs, their children must discern what they are obligated to do and how to balance their obligations to parents with the compelling competing responsibilities, including work, children, and partners. Whose quality of life takes precedence [is difficult to determine] in this harrowing juggling act."[4] This quote by Rabbi Dayle Friedman illustrates what makes this role for adult children so challenging. Caregiving comes on top of the personal and professional stressors that are a part of daily life. For example:

- You may be working to support yourself and or your family.
- You may have lost your job and are financially struggling to meet your own needs, let alone the needs of your elder parents.

- You may be one of what I call the "double-decker sandwich genera-tion," finding yourself caught between caring for your own chil-dren and also caring for your parents or even grandparents.
- You are constantly doing and going, believing that more is better and that enough is never enough.

There are many aspects of caregiving to be mindful of and the follow-ing are some of the most common challenging issues for adult children caregivers.

Generational Differences

> "I never really imagined what it would truly be like taking care of my mother. I wonder if I will have the physical and emotional energy to keep doing this and for how long."
>
> —A daughter

As was the case with spouses, caregiving can be influenced by genera-tional differences, and these differences can wreak havoc on you as a caregiver. It is common when caring for Traditionalists to encounter re-sistance, because elders in this generation hold certain expectations and ideas about how you, as the adult child, *should* take care of them. Their expectations and ideas often don't match yours, and for whatever rea-sons, you may find yourself feeling guilty if you don't adhere to their expectations of how care should be provided. Your role as caregiver can easily become consumed by thoughts such as "I should," "I ought to," or "I am not doing enough." All three of these can lead to caregiver resent-ment, overwhelming stress, and caregiver burnout. I share with adult children the following mantra: "Thou shall not should on thyself!" While many of you might at first find this funny, it is a very important mantra to keep in mind. Being a mindful caregiver helps you recognize what *you can and can't* provide. You learn how to set clear boundaries and at the same time find ways to validate and honor these generational differences. Later on, you will learn how to let go of your "shoulds," your "oughts," and the "not doing enough" thoughts.

Role Changes: Is It a Role Reversal or Role Change?

Does the following statement sound familiar? "It feels like I have be-come the parent and my parent has become my child." One of the most upsetting and confusing aspects of caring for an elder parent is when your roles as adult children and parents appear to be reversing. Many call this *role reversal*. Gerontologists suggest that when you believe that your roles reverse, it can demean the elder and doesn't consider all the emotions that accompany this phenomenon for you and your care recipi-ent. In my work with caregivers, I believe that accepting role reversal is neither healthy nor true. Instead, recognize the differences between *role reversal* and *role change.*

Role change occurs when two adults experience a change in their relationship because the ill or incapacitated adult is now dependent on the adult who is well. When this change occurs, there is a shift in roles between the two adults. Role change can bring forth a plethora of feelings, such as sadness, anger, disappointment, and loss. One of the reasons adult caregivers wrestle emotionally with caring for a parent is that it's painful to acknowledge that your roles are changing. It's important to process these emotions, especially when you are caring for someone who has a long-term illness. In addition, adult children often grieve because their "parent" is no longer able to "parent" because of his incapacity. Said another way, your parent is no longer able to share his beliefs, advice, or support in the way you were used to throughout your life. This change can be overwhelming. Your grief can be a harsh reminder that you will eventually lose the care recipient. Identifying and honoring these feelings as you experience the various losses with your care recipient can help you learn to cope more effectively. (Chapter 8 provides more information on grieving.)

While adult children certainly face role changes throughout the caregiving journey, there can also be *role opportunities.* Let me share an example as the best way to define what is meant by this. When my mother was diagnosed with Alzheimer's disease, I was thirty-five years old. I had been accustomed to having my mother's guidance and support all those years. I knew that with Alzheimer's disease, my mother would continue to decline physically and cognitively. Knowing that chronic illness can cause changes in roles and relationships, I wanted to find ways to continue to maintain our roles as mother and daughter for as long as possible. I was not willing to fall victim to the belief that role reversal takes place. This meant that *I* had to make many adjustments, as my mother could not. I wanted to find *opportunities* for us to relate as mother and daughter.

I will never forget my experience with my mother when my father died. By then, my parents had been divorced about thirty years and my mother's dementia was pretty significant. Her short-term memory was quite impaired, she had trouble completing sentences, and she relied on a wheelchair for mobility. After my father's funeral, I felt a great need to have my mother comfort and mother me. When Mom saw me get off the elevator, her face brightened. After we exchanged hellos, I told her that I had something important to share, that her ex-husband, Danny, had died, and that I had just returned from his funeral. She sat quiet for a minute, then turned to me and said, "Good for him." Her comment took me by surprise and I sort of smiled. But then, I turned toward her and said, "Mom, I know you and Dad are divorced and that you didn't have a good relationship with him, but he still was my father and I feel sad that he died." The next thing I knew, my mother reached out to me with both her hands, from her wheelchair, to pull me close to her so she could hug me. I started crying and she just held me. In that special moment, she was my mother, and I was her child who needed comforting. I share this experience because it reinforces that by my giving my mother an opportunity to be "my mother" despite her dementia, she was able to rise to the occasion. Throughout my mother's illness, I chose to find these role opportunities. I tried to stay connected to my mother and communicate with her about aspects of my life and her life until the very end of her disease. Truthfully, I am not sure how much she was able to understand. What mattered was that I could continue to treat her as my mother and honor our mother–daughter relationship.

As I have said many times now, each caregiver journey is unique. I recognize not all caregivers will be interested or able to discover new role opportunities. Yet, for those who are able to do so, the gifts you can receive are immeasurable.

When to Step In and Make Decisions for the Care Recipient

> "How do I respect my mother's wishes to be independent, and at the same time step in because she is heading down a path of self-destruction by drinking herself to death?"
>
> —A desperate daughter-caregiver

Another area of great concern for many adult children caregivers is figuring out when to step in and make decisions for your parents. When should you move them, take over their finances, or tell them they can't drive anymore? How do you determine if your parent is competent or not? Who else should be involved in decision making, and how do you decide who takes the lead? Determining when to take over for another adult is one of the most gut-wrenching decisions adult children can face. Making decisions for a parent or older adult can elicit an avalanche of mixed emotions. Most adult children caregivers are often reluctant to make decisions for their care recipient because they don't want to take away their independence. Our culture values independence as one of the most important virtues of being an adult. As such, we're expected to be able to take care of ourselves and be in control of our lives. Ironically, the desire to be independent (our way of saying we don't want to be a burden) is often what creates the biggest burden for caregivers.

I recall a common situation that speaks to the "when to take over" issues between adult children and elder care recipients. An adult son, Ken, was struggling with how to take over his mother's finances. His mother had dementia and still believed she should be in charge. Whenever he attempted to convince her he needed to take over, she would yell at him and say, "You are treating me like a child and trying to take over my life." On one occasion when Ken was visiting his mother, he happened to see a number of pieces of unopened mail dated months earlier. As he opened each letter, he found out that his mother was not paying many of her bills and was accruing enormous finance charges. This prompted him to get in touch with me. When I had asked Ken how he had attempted to take over his mother's finances, he sheepishly shared the following: "Frankly, I couldn't stand listening to her yell and berate me each time I tried to talk with her about her finances. So I just gave in. Yet, now we are in one heck of a mess." It took Ken months to clear up all the debt. And with my support and coaching, Ken was able to take a stand with his mother and most importantly *not personalize* her accusations. He had to acknowledge that her dementia was interfering with her ability to be independent. Addressing the issues of independence takes a lot of courage and a certain amount of finesse, for sure. This next section takes a closer look at how to navigate through this often very treacherous terrain.

CAREGIVERS AND COMPETENCY

The topic of competency is fraught with challenges and discomfort. Determining competency is not easy. And it is important to understand how the law defines competency when an adult is ill. The most critical question when determining competency is whether your care recipient is *cognitively or psychologically* impaired. The following points can help you begin to assess whether you have a competency issue.

Does your care recipient:

- Have the ability to analyze or process information?
- Understand his current medical situation?
- Recognize that she is utilizing poor judgment and insight?
- Understand when his safety may be in jeopardy, such as when driving a car, using the stove, or taking medications?
- Have significant depression that is impairing her ability to make decisions?
- Have concentration challenges, such as having difficulty following conversations, reading books, or watching movies?

If your answers indicate a problem or are unsure about how to answer these questions, then by all means have your care recipient seen by a professional. A geriatric physician, geriatric psychiatrist, neuropsychologist, or geriatric social worker can provide appropriate evaluations and help you to determine competency. Some of the more complicated situations may require legal and medical intervention. If this describes your situation, I would highly encourage you to also contact an attorney specializing in guardianship matters or elder care law.

When it is *clear* that your care recipient is *unable* to make informed decisions and you have his power of attorney (POA), you will need to invoke it. (A POA is described in detail in chapter 8 but basically means that you have the legal authority to make decisions on behalf of your care recipient. Your care recipient, at some point, would have had to sign legal documents that gave you the right to be the POA.) You may feel uncomfortable with stepping in, but it is critical to do so. It is the best way to make sure your care recipient is well cared for and to prevent a crisis from occurring. If you have a care recipient who is resisting help, you may need professional help to move forward. Later in this section, I provide some case examples of how to navigate through this very trying aspect of caregiving.

When caregivers *don't* have power of attorney and your care recipient is *not competent*, then you will most likely have to apply for *guardianship*. Guardianship is a matter of state law and varies from jurisdiction to jurisdiction. Guardianship allows a person chosen by the court to act on your care recipient's behalf. You can petition the court to be your care recipient's guardian. Guardianship requires legal intervention. The process takes time and can be fairly costly. Once you become a guardian, you are held responsible by the court. There is significant court oversight, in particular if you are managing your care recipient's finances. For guardians of finances, the guardian would have to file an annual report with the probate court of all the expenditures. For guardians of the person, there is an annual short form that advises the court of exactly where the care recipient is residing and about his general medical conditions and needs. These were put into place to guard against someone taking advantage of an incompetent person. However, it does give you full power to transact business and make health-care decisions for your care recipient—just realize it provides additional work for caregivers.

In extreme situations—when your care recipient is resisting help and is unsafe—you can either contact your local Adult Protective Services Department to investigate the situation or apply for an *emergency temporary guardianship*. Note that many different states call this department by different names, including Office on Aging and Adult Services, Department of Family and Protective Services, or Elderly Protective Services. Let me explain how each works.

If you decide to call protective services, you will be asked a series of questions, including why you believe your care recipient is in harm's way. Generally speaking, protective services will not investigate unless they believe there is either immediate danger to the care recipient or another person. Immediate danger means that there is a significant chance your care recipient (or another person) will be hurt from the current situation. In order to assess the situation further, protective services will visit the home and make their own determination. If they conclude your care recipient is in imminent danger, they will make recommendations about the type of care or placement your care recipient needs. Oftentimes, a case worker will be assigned to ensure the plan is carried out.

I recommend to caregivers that you reserve this as an intervention of last resort.

The second type of last-resort intervention is to obtain an emergency temporary guardianship. Again, the law on this issue varies from jurisdiction to jurisdiction. Generally the law provides a procedure for obtaining temporary guardianship on an expedited or emergency basis if the situation is dire and there is an immediate and substantial risk of death or serious physical injury. Temporary guardianship is usually effective for sixty days with the understanding that during that time frame the guardian will undertake the steps necessary to become the permanent guardian of the care recipient. This process involves filing a petition with the local probate court and then appearing to give testimony before the probate judge. It does, however, allow you immediate legal authority to place your care recipient—even against his wishes—into a hospital, assisted living, or nursing home for a stated period of time to ensure that your care recipient is safe. Both of these interventions can place you in very uncomfortable situations. However, if you don't move forward and take action, a crisis could occur with tragic results.

The following examples illustrate the complexity of competency issues.

"You Have to Convince My Mother That She Needs Help!"—Claire and Her Mother, Kathy

One of the first client families in my private practice involved an elder woman, Kathy, who had Parkinson's disease. Kathy had been living alone in her condo for more than twenty years. Her daughter, Claire, hired me to "convince her mother" that she should have a full-time caregiver. Kathy had recently fallen several times, but luckily hadn't yet broken any bones or hurt herself badly enough to be hospitalized. I assured Claire that I would do my best to evaluate Kathy's situation and make some recommendations.

After meeting Kathy, it was evident that her Parkinson's disease was significant and causing problems. Her balance and walking were impaired enough that she needed a walker. Kathy admitted that she was falling more. Kathy also had considerable tremors, which made tying shoes, buttoning blouses, and opening containers difficult. However, she somehow was managing. Cognitively, Kathy was competent and sharp. When I asked her questions regarding her safety and need for help, Kathy clearly said to me, "Nancy, I know I am an accident waiting to happen, but I also am a very private person. I am not interested in having anyone live with me, nor am I interested in moving into a retirement community." Kathy was adamant about her feelings and seemed to understand the risks involved.

When I reconvened with Claire, I told her I had to go along with her mother's decision. Claire was aghast. My professional belief was that as long as her mother was competent, she had the right to make her own choices, even if they were "lousy ones" or placed her "at risk." Truth be told, many of us make decisions that could impact our health and safety and that is our personal right. While I agreed with Claire that having a caregiver would be the better choice for Kathy, this was not what Kathy wanted. I encouraged Claire to clearly express her disagreement and, at the same time, (unhappily) honor her mother's decision not to hire a caregiver. In addition, I also suggested that Claire needed to let her mother know that her mother would have to be responsible for the consequences of her choices. Lastly, I suggested Claire revisit this topic again, maybe a month or so later. Although this was not the way Claire had hoped things would have worked out, she realized she had to let go. And, of course, this is especially difficult when you believe the decision made by the elder is not in her best interests. In this situation, the irony of it all was that about four weeks later, Kathy had a massive stroke and survived the stroke. Now things had changed dramatically. Kathy was not competent and Claire would have to make all the decisions for Kathy. The moral of this story is that sometimes no one has control.

A Case of Hoarding—One Family's Struggle to Help Their Parents

Ted and Martha had been married for fifty-five years and still resided in their home. They had three children who lived in different parts of the country. Martha had been diagnosed with dementia five years earlier; she had no short-term memory and her reasoning and judgment were quite impaired. Martha had a lifetime hobby of attending garage sales. As she aged, her garage-sale buying became an obsession. Then she started to become cognitively impaired and her collecting of things turned into hoarding. Almost every room in their house was filled to the brim with stuff. Ted began feeling overwhelmed. Yet, while he wanted to hire live-in help, Martha was adamantly opposed. Because of Martha's strong personality, Ted felt powerless and reached out to his children for support.

Ted's children contacted me as they too were alarmed at the condition of their parents' home and the stress their father was under. After making a home visit, I recommended a home care agency that could slowly clean out some of the rooms in their house and help Martha with some light housekeeping and cooking. At first, Martha accepted the caregiver help. However, as time went on, this proved to be a very challenging situation. Martha continually complained about the cost and was adamant that they didn't need a caregiver. Midway through this process, Ted fired the home care agency, saying that it was too expensive. After hearing that

Ted fired the home care agency, I encouraged his children to back off for a month or so, and then reevaluate their parents' situation.

I present this case example for several reasons. In this situation, although Martha may have been incompetent, she was married to Ted, who was competent. As a married couple, the competency issue rests on whether one of the parties is still competent. The adult children had to acknowledge that their father was still competent and thus could remain in charge. The key was making sure that their father was not neglecting or placing his wife in danger. While this might not have been the desired outcome for the adult children, a court most likely would have ruled that Ted was not neglectful and, as Martha's husband, could continue to care for her.

"I Can Take Care of My Husband: There Is Nothing Wrong with Me" — A Guardianship Situation

Marilyn asked for a consult regarding her mother, Jessica, who was seventy years old, married, and an active alcoholic living with her third husband, Tom. Jessica and Tom had been married for fifteen years. Marilyn was an only child and Tom had no children. Tom has dementia and Jessica had been caring for him for the past two years. As Tom's dementia became worse, Jessica's drinking increased. On several occasions, Jessica drove over to Marilyn's house while intoxicated. Additionally, Marilyn had become very concerned that Jessica was not taking good care of Tom. She was forgetting to give him his medications and had been neglecting his hygiene. Whenever Marilyn approached Jessica about the situation, Jessica staunchly denied anything was wrong and stated it was none of her business.

After consulting with me, Marilyn and I decided to first try an intervention that involved getting help for Jessica. I went over to her home and asked Jessica to consider placing her husband in an assisted living facility, which could be good for him and help relieve Jessica of some stress. She liked the idea and agreed to check a few out. Several months later, she had not done anything. Marilyn called me again, stating the situation with Jessica and her husband had come to a head, with Tom having a very difficult time communicating and even keeping his balance when walking. Jessica was drinking at an all-time high. It was apparent that Jessica was clearly neglecting her husband and herself.

Unfortunately, the only option was to petition the court for an emergency guardianship, as Marilyn didn't have a POA for her mother. The court granted Marilyn an emergency guardianship, which allowed her to set up an intervention for her mother. At my recommendation, she called the hospital I thought would be best for her mother and explained her intervention plan to the admitting psychiatrist and admissions team. She also had to make sure they would have a bed available. She then had to contact the police department and describe the situation to them. She explained that her plan was to catch her mother driving while intoxicated, which was easy to do as her mother often drove drunk when getting her stepfather. Fortunately, Marilyn was able to call the police while Jessica was drunk and picking up her husband. The police drove Jessica directly to the hospital where she was admitted under temporary guardianship. Now if this weren't enough, Marilyn also had to secure a caregiver for her stepfather while her mother was in the hospital. I was able to help her with that. In extreme situations such as this, there is no way to avoid the incredible stress that comes with getting emergency guardianship and dealing with the circumstances. Whenever possible, try to get help and support from a professional.

Therapeutic Lying

As caregivers can see, competency issues are not the easiest. However, when your care recipient is incompetent due to cognitive impairment, dementia, serious depression, or alcohol or drug abuse, you must find a way to step in and take over. In my work with caregivers, one of the most effective ways to help for your care recipient is to utilize a strategy called *therapeutic lying*. Hearing the word *lying* may cause some of you to feel a bit uncomfortable. However, let me provide some insight to help you understand its utility. Therapeutic lying involves creating a "white lie" in order to provide an opportunity for professional intervention. The goal of the therapeutic lie is to help the care recipient without creating too much trauma for everyone involved. In essence, the approach helps move the care recipient into a safer and more appropriate situation. It is important to point out that therapeutic lying should be used only when there is a safety concern and resistance from the care recipient, coupled with cognitive impairment.

I have successfully utilized therapeutic lying in many difficult caregiving situations. It requires careful consideration and thoughtful planning. In most cases, this intervention should be used in tandem with a professional who can help you develop the therapeutic lie and the implementation plan. Let me provide a few examples of how therapeutic lying can be effective.

"I Am Not Moving" — Mathew and His Mother, Lillian

Lillian was an eighty-five-year-old woman who had dementia. Her husband of fifty years had died suddenly from a stroke. Not wanting his mother to be by herself, Mathew moved his mother into his home while he and his wife could determine the best place for her. Mathew knew Lillian had some short-term memory problems, but he didn't realize how progressive her dementia had become until Mathew's father died. After living with them for about a month, Mathew recognized that his mother would not be safe to return to her home without professional caregiver help. In deference to her, Mathew and his wife told Lillian that they would like to hire a caregiver to help out when she returned home. They hoped she would agree. However, Lillian completely denied needing help, insisting she could return to her home by herself. She emphatically stated, "I will not have anyone else in my home living with me except your father." When Mathew reminded Lillian that her husband was no longer alive, she stated that her neighbors would help and that she'd be "just fine." Lillian's son and daughter-in-law felt powerless and reluctantly let Lillian move back into her home by herself.

Within a few days, it was clear that Lillian was not "just fine." She called them several times a day and asked the same questions over and over. Even though they delivered meals and created reminders for her medications, Mathew noticed that Lillian was not taking her medications correctly and wasn't eating the food. Mathew and his wife knew that it was not safe for Lillian to live alone. Plus, Lillian would not allow caregiver help in her home. Their only option was to place Lillian in assisted living care. Knowing that Lillian would refuse to leave, Mathew contacted me.

My first hurdle in helping this family was to figure out how to make a home visit without Lillian becoming anxious or suspicious about why I was visiting, hence the first therapeutic lie. The therapeutic lie involved telling Lillian that I was from her homeowners' association and was conducting a survey of her condo unit. The goal of the therapeutic lie would be to evaluate her and her home without Lillian feeling too uncomfortable. I accomplished both in just over an hour. She felt comfortable with me, and I was able to make an assessment. The assessment confirmed that she was not only experiencing significant dementia but also was quite depressed. Moving Lillian into assisted living where she would have twenty-four-hour supervision, medical support, and socialization would be the best choice.

The next hurdle was to figure out how to move her, knowing that Lillian would be very resistant. I suggested returning to the condominium and telling her a second therapeutic lie. This therapeutic lie involved telling Lillian that her condominium association was requiring an update to her unit's electrical system, which would require her to move out for a few days. I informed her that the condominium management company made arrangements for the tenants to temporarily move into another apartment. Although Lillian was not thrilled about this situation, she agreed to move. The temporary apartment was in the assisted living community. When she realized where she was, she became upset. However, with the support of the professional staff, she made the adjustment quite well. She made new friends, and her emotional and physical health improved. However, each time Mathew would visit Lillian, she would continually complain about living there and ask to go home. With coaching from me, Mathew and his wife learned how to address this issue. They were able to distract Lillian and over time, their visits became quite pleasant. The move into assisted living, while not easy, was important for Lillian's safety. And an important benefit for Mathew and his wife was decreased stress and worry, and increased ease. In this situation, the only way we could have moved Lillian forward without a crisis or traumatic event was utilizing the therapeutic lie.

"Once a Doctor, Always a Doctor" — Family Caregivers and Earl, Care Recipient

Another example of utilizing the therapeutic lie involved a man, Earl, who was seventy-one, widowed, and a retired physician. He had been diagnosed with Alzheimer's disease (AD) about ten years earlier. Earl had two daughters and two sons. He also had two sisters with whom he was quite close. He owned one home that he had shared with his wife, and another home in a golf community. Earl was well known in his home community both professionally and personally. He was in denial that he had any cognitive issues. At the point in which I became involved, he was living with one of his sisters. Earl continually asked her when he would be leaving and moving back into his home. His sister struggled with what to say to him. She felt terribly guilty and sad. This family was at their wits' end. He was still driving and at times getting lost. However, both of his sisters felt he should live in his home with professional caregiver help. When the other sister approached him with the idea of moving back into his home with a caregiver, he blatantly stated, "Hell no! I don't need that."

Earl's daughter contacted me because she felt it was time to move him into an assisted living facility. Earl was described by all as fiercely independent, controlling, and stubborn. Earl underwent cognitive testing, which showed that the executive functioning areas of his brain were impaired. His ability to appropriately reason, analyze, and understand was quite impacted by his dementia, and that was on top of his strong personality. I felt quite certain Earl was going to be resistant to any professional help.

In order for me to conduct an assessment and move this family forward, I decided to utilize the therapeutic lie. In this case, I asked one of Earl's physician colleagues to help. His colleague introduced me as a real estate agent who could help Earl find a golf community near his hometown where he could retire. (Hence the therapeutic lie.) Earl was quite gracious when talking with me, yet I could tell that convincing him to move was not going to be easy. Throughout the interview, Earl would digress from the discussion about the golf community and repeatedly state that he wanted to go back to his own home. He didn't understand why his family was so concerned about him. At the end of our time together, he adamantly insisted that he "would go home, whether his family liked it or not."

In this situation, Earl was very resistant and unaware of his cognitive deficits. While my therapeutic lie allowed me to conduct an evaluation, the family had to take it one step further. Since Earl would not give anyone POA, the only way to place him into an assisted living/dementia care community was for his family to obtain temporary guardianship — which they got. This allowed his family to get him admitted to a geriatric psychiatric hospital. The hospitalization helped stabilize him and adjust his medications. We then thoughtfully planned how he would be moved to an assisted living community. Ultimately, with some careful transition work, I was able to match him to a facility with experience in handling resistance and his type of dementia. This community looked like a golf community as well, which helped him settle in more easily. Over time, Earl declined physically as well as medically and he required nursing home care. Because he still related a great deal to being a doctor, I knew that an important aspect of easing him into the nursing home community was to create a "job" so that he felt needed. I suggested that the staff ask him to help chart the medical care of the residents. They provided him with "made up" charts he could review. Everyone in the nursing home calls him Doc. Unfortunately, Earl's disease has progressed. Yet despite his significant dementia, he thinks he is the director of the place and he continues to review charts and tell the nurses what to do.

"No One Can Keep Up with Us" — Selma and George

I received a frantic call from Anne, who was extremely concerned about her parents, both of whom had dementia. They have been married for fifty years, did everything together, and were living in their own home. Although numerous doctors had recommended that George no longer drive, each of the doctors was fired immediately after that recommendation. The fact that George was still driving, despite being told otherwise, terrified Anne and her brother. Additionally, Anne's mother, Selma, was experiencing hallucinations and paranoia, both of which were not treated. And because both of them suffered from impaired short-term memory, they were not appropriately taking their medications. They were in pretty good physical shape and were very proud that they walked several miles a day, even bragging that "no one could keep up with them." Neither George nor Selma recognized that each had memory issues.

I made my first home visit with the therapeutic lie that I was a representative from the hospital where the wife had had hip surgery. My goal was to establish a relationship, help bring in home care, and prevent George from driving. In talking with them, it was clear that Selma was in charge and her husband agreed with whatever she said. When the session was over, they seemed comfortable with me and even invited me back. My next step was to get them to a geriatric doctor so that they both could be evaluated appropriately. I suggested their most trusted son recommend a new doctor. So the second therapeutic lie involved having the son tell his parents that he really liked his new doctor and wanted them to meet him. They agreed to see the doctor and because we all discussed the approach in advance, the doctor won their trust.

The third therapeutic lie involved strategizing on how to best get them into an assisted living facility. The doctor and I decided to focus on George. During the appointment, the doctor told them that George's new heart medication would require careful monitoring by a nurse. His choice was to either go into the hospital or into an assisted living community. Knowing that Selma would not want to be separated from George, they reluctantly agreed to go into the assisted living community. At their appointment with me, I reinforced the choice by stressing that Selma could be with George and even sleep in the same bed. I hoped that their behavior, mood, and cognition might improve because they would be eating better and taking their medication properly. I also was interested in finding out how they would get along with the caregivers, as this would help me assess how to bring a caregiver into their home. Getting the proper medications helped tremendously. While George did quite well with the caregivers, Selma was not happy, nor did she appreciate the caregivers. Selma, however, was concerned about her husband, so both the doctor and I thought we might be able to pull off the next intervention.

The fourth therapeutic lie involved the doctor saying that their insurance would pay for a caregiver so we could get them back home. The doctor indicated that it would be important for the caregiver to monitor George's vital signs and cook special meals for him. Desiring to get back to their home, they agreed. I found a caregiver who could keep up with them, and even walk daily. At first they balked at the caregiver coming every day, but after she kept up with them during the first walk, they bragged about her. The caregiver even coined a name to call themselves—"the fast pacers." I share this situation to point out that some situations are quite challenging and require professional help and support.

I hope these examples provide insight and knowledge about how to successfully keep your care recipient safe. There is no doubt that competency issues are challenging. Letting go of the outcome is difficult. It takes tremendous courage and a willingness to be open to a variety of approaches. If you keep an open mind and heart, your caregiving journey can be easier, and you may even be able to find some humor and blessings along the way.

VALIDATING YOUR ROLE AS A MINDFUL CAREGIVER

Caregivers deserve to be recognized as heroes for all the lives they have saved and save.

I close this chapter by saying thank you to all who have cared endlessly for their care recipient, sacrificed their own health and well-being, placed their lives on hold, and trudged through the muck and yuck of being a caregiver. Being a caregiver can be a thankless job. And while most of you don't become caregivers out of a need to be recognized, *validating* all you do and have done deserves *recognition* and *appreciation*. For many, caregiving is an intimate experience laced with sadness, difficulty, embarrassment, and unglamorous tasks. As a result, many caregivers tend to keep their roles very private. As such, family members and friends may have no clue what is involved. I believe that this role deserves highlighting so that more people in our society will lend support, show more compassion, and offer successful role models. The caregivers I have met over the years are amazing people. Most do whatever it takes to provide the best care possible for their care recipient. And a good many take on this role under very difficult circumstances. Caregivers can be the worst at acknowledging their great qualities and positive attributes. It's important to remind them of their value and how well they perform their roles.

Acknowledging Caregiver Values and Qualities

My guess is that the majority of caregivers will be able to identify with the following values and qualities. As you read through this list, take a moment to reflect on how these words feel to you. Breathe them in one word at a time, and then let them float into your heart.

Generous, courageous, patience, dedicated, caring, accepting, flexible, kind, gentle, loving, compassionate, strong, honest, thoughtful, willing, attentive, assertive, bold, organized, witty, warm, open minded, resilient, empathetic, aware, hopeful, faithful, responsible, tolerant, insightful, joyful, daring, unflappable, fair, passionate, unique, efficient, heartful, humble, productive, fearless, helpful, supportive, altruistic, collaborative, cooperative, grateful, articulate, attentive, considerate, sensitive, observant, powerful, respectful, adaptable, proactive, insightful intelligent. . .

Next, choose a word from the list (or use another one) and let that word guide your day. For example, if you choose the word "warm," consider how you can find warmth in all aspects of your role as caregiver. Perhaps you wrap yourself in warm feelings or value the warmth of the caregiver who helps support your care recipient. Staying mindful of the positive attributes you bring to this role can help you appreciate yourself.

Honoring Your Role as Caregiver

In the beginning of this chapter, I mentioned that there are many different ways caregivers enter into the role of caregiver. I believe being a caregiver to a frail person is a pretty serious position to hold—yet I am not sure that our culture sees it that way. Interestingly, we honor various roles and professions in our culture, such as mothers, fathers, teachers, and secretaries, yet while there now is a National Caregivers day, most people are not aware of it and it's hardly mentioned by the media. There are no cards thanking caregivers for the amazing care they provide. Hopefully, at some point in the near future, caregivers will receive not only the recognition they deserve but also the financial and emotional support they need. Mindful caregivers know and always keep in their hearts that "they matter."

Recognizing Your Own Growth as a Caregiver

Last but not least, it can be very rewarding for you to be aware of how you have grown through the caregiving journey. Sometimes it takes having some distance from your role to truly be able to see how you have evolved. As mindful caregivers, I encourage you to stay conscious of these incredible life lessons and growth opportunities. In my work with caregivers, many have shared how they grew from the experience of being a caregiver. For example:

- They learned to appreciate some of their own qualities and virtues.
- They were able to develop new sides of themselves, such as more self-confidence and self-esteem.
- They learned how to trust their intuition.
- They learned new skills they either never had or didn't have the confidence to do.
- They made new friends and treasured grace moments.
- They learned how to value and appreciate what they had.
- They became more aware of the blessings in their lives.
- They learned to value the little things and little moments.
- They found meaning and become more introspective. They learned to flex different character muscles, such as patience, flexibility, open-mindedness, gratitude, and compassion.
- They felt stronger and more empowered.

I leave you with a final thought: Being a caregiver teaches you how to "dance in the rain." You may experience plenty of rain and storms throughout your caregiving journey. Yet most caregivers find that when the rain or storms slow down or stop, they are usually followed by sunshine and perhaps even a rainbow.

NOTES

1. Centers for Disease Control and Prevention and the Kimberly-Clark Corporation, "Assuring Healthy Caregivers, a Public Health Approach to Translating Research into Practice: A Re-Aim Framework" (2008).

2. Marty Richards, *Caresharing: A Reciprocal Approach to Caregiving and Care Receiving in the Complexities of Aging, Illness or Disability* (Woodstock: SkyLight Paths, 2009).

3. Barbara Okun and Joseph Nowinski, *Saying Goodbye: How Families Can Find Renewal through Loss* (New York: Penguin Group, 2011).

4. Dayle A. Friedman, *Jewish Visions for Aging: A Professional Guide for Fostering Wholeness* (Woodstock: Jewish Lights, 2008), 96.

TWO

Realistic Expectations

Whose Need Is It Anyway?

We can be so focused on a specific goal that we fail to notice that the solution to our problem cannot be found on the path we have been so feverishly pursuing.

—Naomi Levy, *To Begin Again*, 198

Caring for someone who has a chronic illness, particularly someone with dementia, is a commitment that can last many years. Approaching this challenge realistically is critical to maintaining overall health and well-being. Unfortunately, I have found that many caregivers tend to hold onto *unrealistic expectations*.

Unrealistic expectations are beliefs that you hold that are not feasible, practical, or even achievable. These beliefs are often accompanied with statements telling yourself what you "must," "should," or "have to" do as a caregiver. For example, I often hear caregivers say, "I should be doing more." Caregivers tend to struggle with what the care recipient *desires* versus what the care recipient *needs*. Being *realistic* requires setting aside your personal feelings so that you can pay attention to the *needs* of your care recipient. It also requires making sure you are realistic about what you truly can provide without jeopardizing your own health. This is not easy. The following three examples offer new ways to set realistic expectations so you take better care of yourself.

"If Only I Could Please My Mother"—From a Daughter's Perspective

"If only I could just figure out how to please my mother. What I do for her is never enough!"

Amy consulted me because she was continually frustrated and angry with her demanding mother. Amy was an only child, and throughout her life she was expected to always be available to her mother. Amy felt that she could never please her mother. No matter what she tried to do, it was never enough. In addition, she and her mother were not close. So when Amy's mother developed Parkinson's disease, her mother expected her to be available to help her whenever she needed her. It seemed that whenever Amy planned to go out of town, her mother's Parkinson's disease symptoms would become worse. Amy struggled with whether she should go out of town or not. Most of the time, her guilt would win out, and she would end up canceling her trip so she could be there for her mother. She had canceled several trips, which caused great stress between Amy and her husband. In addition, Amy's mother was jealous that Amy spent time with her own children. She often accused Amy of not caring about her and putting them first. Amy was angry and overwhelmed by her mother's demands but unable to say no and set limits. "I feel guilty if I don't do what she wants, yet I resent having to do everything she wants me to do," Amy said.

Learning more about their relationship, it became clear that Amy was unconsciously hoping that if she did what her mother wanted, her mother would finally appreciate her. So Amy kept placing herself in situations where her mother continued to badger her and she remained angry, frustrated, and depleted. This was "their dance." Applying mindfulness meant helping Amy become *aware* that their dance focused only on her mother and not Amy. Amy needed to get in touch with what she needed. This required that Amy not automatically respond to her mother but instead step back and identify her needs. Once Amy started to apply mindfulness, she was able to more readily listen to her heart. Unless her mother was willing to change (and she was not), Amy would need to be the one who changed.

There is no doubt that deeply ingrained patterns are not easy to change. In truth, only *you* can change your own dance steps. In this story, Amy recognized that she would need to change the dance. This involved letting go of her *unrealistic expectations* about what a caregiver "should be." And she had to let go of hoping that her mother would appreciate her and all that she was doing. Amy became mindful of new and realistic ways to interact with her mother and yet hold onto herself in the process. I reminded her that the new dance would take some practice and she would have to take it one step at a time.

Together, Amy and I identified three areas in which she held unrealistic expectations and needed new ones. They involved *letting go of her guilt, learning to set limits,* and *learning to say no to her mother.* I asked Amy which might be the easiest to work on first. Amy chose letting go of her guilt. She truly believed she had been a supportive daughter and that her guilt was not completely warranted. Amy became conscious of how her guilt prevented her from taking care of herself. In order for Amy to change her old patterns, she needed "new dance steps." She learned to recognize that guilt was there for a purpose, and that she must gently and compassionately discern what was best to do about her situation. Mindfulness helped guide Amy, opening the doors for envisioning many more options.

The first time Amy was confronted with the old dance, she had to really stay focused, determined to be mindful of what her purpose was, to let go of her guilt and create a new dance step with her mother. There were some missteps along the way, which is normal and reasonable to expect. However, Amy was relentless in her commitment to changing those patterns and creating new steps. As she successfully accomplished each one, she felt empowered, more at ease, and less attached to the old ways with her mother. And best of all, she was able to take trips with her husband.

"Until Death Do Us Part"—From a Spouse's Perspective

"I have lived with my husband for fifty years. How do I tell him he can't live in his own home anymore?"

By the time spouses are referred to me, they're often exhausted, overwhelmed, and depressed. While they knew they needed help and support, asking for help or accepting help seemed to only add to their feelings of guilt and sadness. The following are some of the unrealistic expectations that spouses may hold:

- "My spouse will not let anyone else care for him. He expects me to take care of him."
- "I don't expect that someone else can provide the type of care I believe my wife needs."
- "It's my responsibility."
- "My children/grandchildren are too busy to help me and I don't want to bother them."

A number of spouses who read these statements may believe they are not unrealistic and may hold ever so steadfast to the belief of what they must do to take care of their care recipients. And while some of those beliefs might be partially true, no one person can completely take care of another without depleting much of her own physical, emotional, and spiritual energy.

The following events exemplify how tightly a spouse can hold onto unrealistic expectations. Ted and Anna were in their mid-eighties and had been married for fifty years. Ted's was caring for his wife, Anna, who had severe diabetes and was blind. Ted had a serious heart condition and had already suffered two heart attacks. Ted's adult children contacted me for help. Their father wasn't getting any down time or doing anything to take care of himself. They begged Ted to take their mother to an adult day care program or to at least hire a companion a few days a week. No matter what the family said, Ted always had an excuse as to why he couldn't do what they suggested. They were at their wits' end.

It was clear that Ted was risking his own health in order to care for his wife. He was committed to his marriage oath "whether in sickness or in health, until death do us part." He insisted it was *his job* to take care of his wife. He provided numerous examples of how and why only he could take care of her. Ted would not leave his wife alone and Anna was too frail to go out. As a result, Ted's personal life was on hold. He had no time for friends or to even attend church. But he greatly resisted changing his patterns and expectations.

In talking with Ted, I pointed out all the wonderful ways he was taking care of his wife. I then asked Ted if he would consider changing his expectations of what he should be doing to care for Anna "just a little." Would he be willing to periodically allow a family or church member to help out? I expressed my concern that his nonstop care was taking a toll on him physically, emotionally, socially, and spiritually. I then asked him what would happen if he had another heart attack and died. For the first time, Ted seemed to understand how he was jeopardizing his own health, which in turn could jeopardize his ability to care for Anna. He agreed, rather hesitantly, to allow a volunteer from his church to stay with his wife for a few afternoons while he took some time for himself. Within a few weeks, Anna took to the volunteer! With encouragement from his family, Ted hired a wonderful companion to stay with his wife two mornings a week. As a mindful caregiver, Ted realized taking good care of himself would allow him to be around to take good care of his wife.

"We Are All in This Together" — From a Family Perspective

I worked with a family in which the father and husband, Jack, had symptoms of Alzheimer's disease but hadn't yet been evaluated by a geriatric physician. In addition, his wife, Louise, was struggling with physical issues that were beginning to wear her down. Louise was particularly stressed out by her husband's denial about his dementia. His forgetfulness was also taking a toll on her. He would repeat himself over and over or ask her the same question right after she had answered him. What really angered her was that she knew Jack needed memory medication but he refused to go to the doctor. Louise was so angry she could barely stand to be in the same room with Jack. Feeling very upset, she turned to her adult children to see if they could help.

Jack's children all strategized about the best approach to get him to the doctor. The family determined that his grandson might be the best person to take him. He rarely refused an opportunity to be with him. The family arranged to have Jack go with his grandson to the doctor and then out to lunch. Jack agreed to go. However, once there, he refused to cooperate with the doctor. He wouldn't answer when the doctor tried to ask him questions from the Mini-Mental Status Exam. (This is a brief cognitive test to assess memory.) Although he was prescribed medication for his memory issues, he told the doctor and he would not take them. The only procedure he consented to was the CT scan, which indicated there was some atrophy of the brain.

When Louise learned how noncompliant Jack had been, she called her children and broke down crying, saying through her tears that she couldn't cope with this situation anymore.

In situations such as this, the initial outcome was not what the family *expected*. Yet, it was a step in the right direction. While it might not sound like an achievement, getting someone with dementia to go to a doctor when he has been refusing to do so is a major accomplishment. Jack did get to the geriatrician, had one diagnostic test, and was prescribed needed medication. In this situation, the family and his wife had to lower their expectations and focus on one step at a time—and recognize the progress that was made. As Rabbi Dayle Friedman shares, "Families sometimes need to measure accomplishment differently. Progress may be in millimeters not inches."[1]

Lastly, I need to highlight an issue that is rarely discussed in the caregiving books. It is when unrealistic expectations can negatively impact the safety and well-being of the care recipient. This can occur because the caregiver has unrealistic expectations about her ability to care for the care recipient. For example, the caregiver may not be physically able to care for the care recipient. Or the caregiver can be so exhausted and overwhelmed that she is not thinking clearly. Or the caregiver may be in denial of how bad the situation has become. Thus, as a result, the care recipient can be unintentionally neglected. These cases tend to be few and far between, but they do take place. For example, if the caregiver is mentally competent and continues to hold unrealistic expectations about the caregiving situation, legal intervention from another adult is necessary, such as emergency guardianship. It is important that the care recipient is removed from harm. These situations can be emotionally difficult for the caregiver and require a great deal of professional support. First steps generally involve enlisting the support of an attorney and the care recipient's physician. These professionals can help everyone navigate through the challenging issues.

As the reader can now see, unrealistic expectations can interfere in a variety of ways and place both the caregiver and care recipient in danger. Let's now look at ways caregivers can become more mindful of what is realistic.

QUESTIONS TO HELP YOU DEVELOP REALISTIC EXPECTATIONS

While setting realistic expectations is not easy, a mindfulness approach can help you sort through the complexities of caregiving so you can proceed as *reasonably* as possible. The questions below are designed to help cultivate awareness and balance. As Paula Reeves suggests in her book *Heart Sense*,[2] it's important to discover ways to get your mind and heart in concert with one another.

Are you willing to:

- Recognize what you can and cannot do and admit to your own limitations?
- Let go of those things you don't have control over?
- Ask for support when you need it, and be clear about what you need?
- Take time to care for yourself?

As you begin to answer these questions, be aware of how your heart and mind are reacting. Be mindful and listen to *your own voice*, not just the voice of your care recipient. Ask what you *can realistically expect* of yourself. When you are realistic, you are more likely to accept what you can and can't do.

Emotions and Caregiving: Riding the Emotional Rollercoaster

> The biggest risk in our daily life is neither stress nor burnout, but numb-out.
>
> —Paula M. Reeves, *Heart Sense*, 107

Holding onto unrealistic expectations can impact you emotionally as well. Your caregiving duties can sometimes be so overwhelming that you don't even *feel* whatever you may be experiencing. When you are constantly busy, you have no time to experience your emotions. Our society sanctions us staying busy. It helps us to remain distant from our pain or from having to acknowledge our situation. We value staying busy and do everything in our power to fill in the gaps—by being on the computer or using our other personal devices, watching television, or doing whatever it takes to distract ourselves from how we are truly feeling.

Don't Be Afraid to Own All Your Feelings

> Clearly recognizing what is happening inside us, and regarding what we see with an open, kind and loving heart, is what is called Radical acceptance.
>
> —Tara Brach, *Radical Acceptance*, 26

Your feelings are vitally important and should not be pushed aside. They are a part of you. Remember, you need to give yourself permission to experience the array of mixed feelings and emotions. Author Tara Brach suggests that sometimes it takes "radical acceptance" when learning to stay with your feelings—good or bad. Applying radical acceptance is a way to hold and accept your feelings and experiences without judgment and a way to gain clarity. Radical acceptance requires that you treat yourself with compassion.[3] In essence, there will be times when you will feel angry, frustrated, guilt ridden, and fearful. You may feel like running away or wish your situation were just a bad dream. Then there will be times when you experience feelings of joy, intense love, and compassion. You may even experience gratefulness for the special time you have with the care recipient. Radical acceptance embraces honoring all your feelings and at the same time recognizing when you need to move on.

In the many years of caring for my mother, it wasn't until I *allowed myself to feel* all my emotions and *gave myself permission* to let some of them go that I was able to appreciate and value my caregiving role. Once I acknowledged my feelings, I was more able to accept the changes that occurred during my mother's illness. It helped me "radically accept" my situation.

The following caregiving example provides you with some ways to acknowledge and cope with your emotions and perhaps apply a radical acceptance approach to your situation.

"When Love Gets in the Way"—From a Spouse's Perspective

Ed's wife, Mabel, had suffered several strokes over the past few years, each one causing her to decline cognitively and physically. When he hired me for a consultation, she was currently living in a rehabilitation center. She had suffered another stroke. This was her second one within three months.

Ed was struggling with whether he should have Mabel stay at the rehabilitation center longer or bring her home and hire home care. Her Medicare rehabilitation benefits were almost depleted, so it was pertinent that a decision on her residence be made soon. Ed expressed his love for his wife and his feelings of confusion about where his wife should live. Although this was a second marriage for both of them, Ed wanted to do everything he could for her. They had both pledged to be at each other's side no matter what. On the one hand, he wanted to take her home, but he was concerned about whether all her medical needs could truly be cared for at home, as Mabel was continuing to have seizures and TIAs (little strokes), was very weak, unable to walk, incontinent, and had episodes of confusion and memory loss. Ed was a competent and caring husband, but he was overwhelmed, exhausted from stress, and confused about the best decision for his wife. He had very mixed feelings. During Mabel's more lucid periods, she expressed her desire and longing to go home. Knowing her desires, Ed was in tremendous emotional pain, struggling to be a good caring husband. And to complicate matters, Mabel's children felt strongly that she should return home and repeatedly pressured Ed to bring her back home. In fact, without telling Ed, Mabel's children had been making arrangements for a hospital bed, wheelchair, home care, and bedside commode so that she could go home. All the emotional stress of the situation was affecting Ed's blood pressure. He was beginning to be concerned about his own health as well.

After conducting the assessment, I suggested Ed consider keeping his wife at the facility for at least the next month until she was more medically stable. Her medical condition was complicated and ever-changing, plus Mabel was on an enormous amount of medications. I also suggested a family meeting with Mabel's adult children and Ed. A meeting was convened; afterwards, it was clear Mabel's children felt their mother had the right to go home if she so desired. They urged their stepfather to take her home. Ed felt pressured by her children, so he gave in and took Mabel home.

After she had been home a few weeks, Ed returned for another consult. He said that the stress of Mabel being home was "killing him." He went on to say his wife had more bad days than good and was often confused. He said he finally realized that he could not realistically keep her at home. I encouraged another family meeting. In this meeting, Ed listened to his voice, stood up for himself, and told the children that he could no longer keep Mabel at home. They became angry with him and refused to speak with him. Although Ed felt badly, he knew he had made the best decision for both himself and his wife. He ended up having Mabel assessed by a hospice, which resulted in her being placed in an inpatient hospice care facility. (Refer to chapter 8, which defines and describes hospice care.) It turned out that Mabel was more ill than her children wanted to acknowledge. Ed joined a spousal support group and set up a few additional sessions with me. He reconnected with his church. This was very important because his church community nourished his spirit, allowing him to be better equipped to show compassion and love to his wife. And because his church offered several different types of fitness programs, he joined a tai chi program and a walking group. Not surprisingly, Ed's blood pressure dropped, he felt less depressed, and began to regain his energy. Ed felt more at ease, and Mabel died at peace in the hospice.

THE CHALLENGES FACED BY NONFAMILY CAREGIVERS

In the caregiving field, little attention has been paid to *nonfamily caregivers*. Yet, as families shrink in size and people live farther away from their families, it becomes necessary for more nonfamily caregivers to provide care. Interestingly, I have found that many nonfamily caregivers place high expectations on themselves as well. They take their role seriously, and as with spouses or family caregivers, they adamantly hang onto their own unrealistic expectations. They believe that since they "volunteered," they can't expect others to help out.

There are additional challenges that nonfamily caregivers may experience. Because nonfamily caregivers don't have the relational history, they don't always know what might be best for the care recipient. Nonfamily caregivers are not always recognized by society as "true family," yet they provide advocacy and care as if they were. Being in this situation can lead to feelings of loneliness and isolation. In addition, many nonfamily caregivers may have their own family members who need attention and support. This can lead to competing demands for time and attention. To help ease their caregiving experience, nonfamily caregivers may want to consider developing a support network around their care recipient. For example, find out if the care recipient belongs to an organization or faith community that could provide some support. Perhaps a college student might be involved or the county has a "friendly visitor" program in the Office on Aging. (Chapter 6 discusses resources and services in-depth.)

Before you commit to becoming a nonfamily caregiver, be mindful of the potential issues that may come with the role. Here's an example.

"What Did I Get Myself Into?" — A Nonfamily Caregiver's Perspective

Sharon and Jane had worked together for many years and had remained friends even after Jane retired. There was a twelve-year age difference between them: Jane was seventy-five, and Sharon was sixty-three. Jane was single and had no family. Fortunately, she had a substantial estate and had been living independently in her condo for more than twenty years. In the past year, Sharon had become concerned about Jane. She noticed that Jane struggled with memory and had problems completing sentences, often mixing words. Jane was in total denial regarding both.

Jane had recently fallen, broken her shoulder, and was in rehabilitative care. After the fall, Sharon began to assist Jane with paying her bills. During that time, Sharon noticed that Jane's checkbook was disorganized and lacked vital information about names and check amounts. Being concerned, Sharon hired me for a consultation. I suggested that Jane see a neurologist. The evaluation showed significant memory issues that included paranoia and deficits in judgment, reasoning, and language—and resulted in a diagnosis of Alzheimer's disease.

Sharon now became the power of attorney (POA) and guardian for her friend. She hired an attorney to help work out the estate details. However, what she didn't realize was the sensitive and difficult decisions she would have to make being the POA for Jane. When Sharon became Jane's POA, one of the major decisions she faced was where Jane would live. Understandably, Jane wished to return to her condominium and

stated she did not need assistance. However, the rehabilitation professionals felt it would be unsafe for her to go back to her condominium
without help. She was not able to understand her needs and limits.

Sharon agonized about what to do. On the one hand, she wondered if
she had the right to not allow her friend to go home, as Jane was demanding this decision. On the other hand, Sharon believed she would be neglecting Jane's safety and well-being if she let her go home. Sharon knew
Jane was a very independent person who liked her privacy. In addition,
Jane tended to be negative and, as a result, didn't trust people and had
few friends. Going back home to her condominium would not be a safe
choice for many reasons. First off, Jane was insistent that she did not need
caregivers and stated that she would fire them. Second, Jane's medical
situation was complicated. She was on a number of medications that
needed to be monitored carefully. Jane simply could not be counted on to
take her medications safely and correctly.

It took great courage for Sharon to hold her ground and move Jane
into assisted living, despite the intense pressure and verbal badgering
from Jane to return to her condo. Jane did not understand why she had to
be moved into the assisted living community and was extremely angry at
Sharon. In addition, Jane was wreaking havoc at the assisted living community, complaining to everyone that Sharon was holding her hostage.
At one point, Jane's behavior upset Sharon so much that she called me in
despair, stating, "I can't believe I am going through all of this when Jane
is not even my family member. I agreed to be her POA because I was
concerned for her and knew she had no one. I did not sign up for this
type of frustration and anger." She stated she was ready to throw in the
towel and let the state find another person to take over for Jane.

Since Jane was so agitated, I suggested a geriatric psychiatric assessment. Jane was assessed and admitted to the hospital so she could be
more closely supervised and have the opportunity to have her medications properly evaluated and titrated. Jane was placed on medication and
began to calm down. She was even able to go back to the assisted living
community. However, not a day passed that Jane didn't ask to go back to
her condominium.

Since Sharon was the sole support for Jane, I encouraged her to create
a "circle of support" so that others could help and support Jane. Sharon
enlisted the support of members of Jane's church, hired a companion to
take Jane on additional outings, and rounded up some former co-workers
to visit. Having the circle of support for Jane not only provided Jane with
needed support, it also helped Sharon not feel overwhelmed from caregiving. Sharon felt tremendous relief and was more at ease knowing she
was not completely responsible for Jane's care.

So let's review the most important points for nonfamily caregivers to
consider. You have to be able to set realistic expectations of what you can
and cannot provide. Look for ways to garner outside support for the care

recipient. Make sure you inform the care recipient's doctor of your limits. Be mindful of overfunctioning or feeling that you are the only one responsible. And keep in mind that sometimes not having the family baggage can actually help you make decisions that can be very positive and meaningful.

RECOGNIZING THAT NOT ALL RELATIONSHIPS ARE HEALTHY

There are some caregiving situations in which the caregivers may not have had a healthy relationship with the care recipient. Caregivers who have been abused, neglected, or harmed by the care recipient need to be mindful about whether they should even provide care. For those who choose *not to provide care*, this decision is not without judgment by others. Our society holds strong expectations that adult children or spouses *should* provide care. In unhealthy relationships, it is critical that you hold onto yourself, no matter what others say or believe.

When a caregiver *chooses to provide care*, the caregiving relationship can be quite challenging and unleash a whole host of feelings and emotions. There can be unfinished business, unresolved feelings, or other issues between caregiver and care recipient that can cause anger, tension, and sadness. While it's always prudent to set limits and boundaries with respect to caregiving, it's especially imperative when the caregiver has suffered abuse or neglect at the hands of the care recipient. In some of the unhealthiest situations, I do not recommend that the adult child or spouse provide direct care to the care recipient. In these situations, I often recommend that caregivers engage the support of a geriatric counselor, clergy professional, or social worker. A professional can help maintain appropriate boundaries, which can be difficult to do on your own. You may need to be involved from a distance, in order to protect and honor your own emotional and spiritual health. Being a mindful caregiver requires you to decide realistically what role, if any, you will assume in the caregiving process. For example, you can make sure that your care recipient is appropriately cared for without having to be directly involved. You can set up appointments with doctors, handle finances, and even pay for certain services. The following examples illustrate these types of relationships and how the caregivers navigated through them.

"This Time Maybe Things Will Be Different"—From the Perspective of an Adult Child Abused by a Parent

Max came to me saying, "We just don't know what to do with our mother." A neighbor had contacted Max and expressed concern about his mother. Her yard was overgrown, the house was in disrepair, and she was behaving very impulsively. He and his siblings had been estranged from their mother, as she had been verbally and emotionally abusive toward them. Feeling obligated to at least find out what was going on, Max decided to visit his mother. When he knocked on her door and shared who he was, she cursed at him and told him to leave. Somehow Max managed to get into the house. Seeing how much his mother had deteriorated, Max immediately contacted his siblings to discuss what they should do. They decided it would be best to consult a geriatric social worker.

After talking with Max, I suggested a family conference call. During this call, each child expressed anger and resentment toward his or her mother. They described stories of being neglected and verbally and emotionally abused, both as children and adults. Even so, they were conflicted about whether they should provide support and care, and to what extent. It was clear that Max and his siblings needed help determining how to set appropriate limits and boundaries. One of her sons shared, "We were hoping that maybe she would soften around the edges, knowing she needed help."

I explained that, unfortunately, their mother had not sought therapy and was just not able to change her interactions with them. In situations such as this, it is necessary to refocus expectations and set limits. It is essential to recognize that feelings of anger, frustration, and sadness are valid and normal. Long-term abuse from a family member makes it extremely difficult to consider helping that person. I told Max and his siblings that if they decided to help, they had to set up strict boundaries ahead of time and that they would need to tell their mother about those boundaries, as well as what behaviors would and would not be tolerated.

Based on Max's most recent experience, I suggested that they consider hiring a mental health professional to advocate for and assess their mother. And if she refused help, they might want to contact Adult Protective Services to intervene. In some circumstances, you may need to find someone else who can represent the other party.

The children did indeed hire an independent professional. Their mother let the professional into her home but was not interested in help for herself. She complained profusely about "how bad" her children were and how they did not care about her. She also tried to talk the professional into contacting her children to get them reengaged in her care. With coaching and support, the children were able to hold their ground. I also talked to the professional and informed her about the reasons Max and his siblings were unwilling to reengage with their mother. While this situation was painful for all, when there is abuse, caregivers have to very mindfully consider their limits and boundaries.

"I Just Can't Do This"—From the Perspective of an Only Child Who Had Been Abused

Charles is another example of someone who had to make caregiving decisions with the backdrop of an abusive history. Charles, who was an only child, found himself thrust into the role of caregiver to his father, who had been physically and verbally abusive to him throughout his life. Charles's father now had cancer and needed help managing his care and his finances. Charles was very clear that he did not want to have any interaction with his father either in person, by phone, or e-mail. Charles had his own financial struggles, and when combined with feelings toward his father, he was unwilling to pay for his father's care. He consulted with me to explore available options for his father. First, I suggested he contact a family services agency that could provide either a care manager or social worker to help his father with his care needs. I also suggested he contact the local cancer organization to find out what resources and services they might be able to provide. Lastly, I mentioned he might contact his father's church to see if they could help out.

Charles did experience some guilt from time to time, but he knew it was the best way to take care of himself. He was mindful that his father needed help and that he did not need to be the only one to provide that help. Charles set realistic expectations for himself; he kept his distance from his father but was able to help provide some care for him through various activities and outlets. People in similar situations should not feel obligated to become caregivers to those who have been abusive. Instead, they can set boundaries and goals that outline the amount of intervention they are willing to make, what level of involvement they will have personally, and how they will go about both helping and *not* helping—when to say "yes" and when to say "no."

Hopefully, the above examples have shed light on the various ways to maintain realistic expectations and boundaries. The bottom line is that each of these situations requires thoughtful consideration. First, caregivers have to get clarity about their own feelings. Next, they have to determine whether they want to become involved. Then, they have to get in touch with what they are willing to do and not do with their care recipient. And most importantly, they have to remember that a mindfulness approach requires compassion about the choices that are made.

POSITIVE ASPECTS OF THE CAREGIVING ROLE: THE GIFTS AND BLESSINGS

> If we become aware and share blessings in our relationships with those we accompany, we will deepen our capacity to be present to all reality.
> —Rabbi Dayle Friedman, *Jewish Visions for Aging*

Many caregivers read the title of this section and wonder how could there be any positive aspects of caregiving for an elder relative. You may ask: "How could there be gifts or blessings when having to care for someone who has Alzheimer's disease or other debilitating chronic ill-nesses?" For some caregivers, there may not be anything positive to be gained from the experience. Yet for some of you, there may be many opportunities in which caregiving can feel rewarding. Caregiving may enhance your own personal growth. There can be gifts and blessings, where laughter and special times can be experienced and cherished.

In my own situation, I learned that the possibility of gifts and bless-ings required that I change my expectations of what could be gained from being one of my mother's caregivers. Doing so helped me appre-ciate and cherish many of the experiences with my mother. I was able to focus on the more positive experiences with my mother, which paved the way for me to cope in a more positive way during the more difficult or sad times.

I realized that there were many gifts and blessings my mother be-stowed upon me in our journey together. I would like to share a few as a way to encourage other caregivers to be open to finding their own. My mother taught me how to be less serious and to laugh more. Often, Mom would try to say one thing and instead a funny mixed-up word or sen-tence would come out. Rather than correcting her, I learned to go with whatever she said. More times than not, it would make both of us laugh because she was still aware of when a word or sentence was not quite right. Mom also taught me to love singing despite not having a great voice (although I can hold a tune). We would lie in bed together and sing away, often making up words to the songs when we couldn't remember them. I learned that at age forty-five it was still okay to lie in bed with her and enjoy our closeness. She taught me the gift of learning to just be. Sitting quietly and sometimes holding her hand brought my mother and me much closer. Most importantly, she taught me that *remembering didn't matter, loving did*. Even when my mother didn't seem to know that I was her daughter, she did know that I loved her. That was the greatest gift of all. To this day, I cherish those gifts and blessings, and they are etched in my heart. I have found that when a caregiver changes her expectations and taps into her spirit, gifts can come forth.

CARE RECIPIENTS' GIFTS AND BLESSINGS

Marty Richards, in her book *Caresharing*, reminds caregivers that they can provide the care recipient with the opportunity to see themselves as "teachers."[4] This thought was also shared in the book *Tuesday's with Morrie*.[5] Morrie struggles with his ALS, a disease that strips away his physical strength and abilities and requires him to be more dependent on others. In Albom's book, he shares how humiliated Morrie felt and kept wondering what he was living for. It isn't until one of Morrie's caregivers shares how much he learned from him about caring for someone that

Morrie sees the gift—he can still be a teacher. He is teaching his caregivers how to care in a compassionate, loving way.

I remember a daughter who shared with me that her mother's illness gave them both a chance to get to know each other better. They spent more time together and appreciated each other so much more since her mother had been diagnosed with cancer. Her mother died feeling her love. She was grateful, as prior to her mother's illness, she had had a difficult time expressing her feelings.

As Dr. Rachel Naomi Remen shares in her book *My Grandfather's Blessings*,[6] "Blessing life moves us closer to each other and closer to our authentic selves. When people are blessed they discover their lives matter, that there is something worthy of blessing. And when you bless others, you may discover this same thing is true about yourself."

My gift to you is that you find your own blessings and moments of grace. I hope this chapter has inspired you to be more realistic with your expectations. I also hope you now feel more empowered to remain open to some of those blessings and gifts into your caregiving journey. Caregiving is an awesome and sacred responsibility. It certainly requires tremendous compassion, patience, and time. The more realistic you can become, the less stress you will experience. This will allow you to focus and harness the energy needed to find ease in your caregiving role.

NOTES

1. Dayle A. Friedman, *Jewish Visions for Aging: A Professional Guide for Fostering Wholeness* (Woodstock: Jewish Lights, 2008), 52.

2. Paula M. Reeves, *Heart Sense: Unlocking Your Highest Purpose and Deepest Desires* (York Beach: Conari Press, 2003), 66.

3. Tara Brach, *Radical Acceptance: Embracing Your Life with the Heart of a Buddah* (New York: Bantam Books, 2003), 26.

4. Marty Richards, *Caresharing: A Reciprocal Approach to Caregiving and Care Recieving in the Complexities of Aging, Illness or Disability* (Woodstock: SkyLight Paths, 2009).

5. Mitch Albom, *Tuesdays with Morrie* (New York: Random House, 1997), 109.

6. Rachel Naomi Remen, *My Grandfather's Blessings: Stories of Strength, Refuge, and Belonging* (New York: Berkley, 2000), 7.

THREE

Self-Care Absolutely Matters!

Self-care is a necessity, not an option. To care for another, you need to care for yourself.

—Marty Richards, *Caresharing*, 22

THE PATH TO BEING A MINDFUL CAREGIVER

How can I take care of myself when all my physical and emotional energy is expended on caring for my loved one? This statement represents an almost universal concern held by caregivers. There is no doubt that, at the end of the day, many caregivers are depleted and exhausted. The idea of having to take care of one more thing, especially themselves, is even more daunting. This chapter focuses on helping caregivers become "mindful caregivers." Mindful caregivers recognize the importance of being *intentional* about the type of care they can realistically provide to the care recipient. They also recognize that they matter too and are dedicated to making sure they take care of themselves. Being intentional requires that caregivers learn to ask themselves the following about how they provide care:

- Is this necessary?
- Am I doing too much?
- Am I expecting too much of myself?

Caring for someone else requires recognizing that if you give and give and don't replenish what you have given, eventually there will be nothing left. The subsequent sections will help caregivers recognize the issues that can get in the way of self-care. I provide ideas, information, and caregiver examples so you can find new ways to take care of yourself.

UNDERSTANDING THE UNIQUENESS OF CAREGIVER STRESS

Many books written about caregiving discuss how caregivers can get rid of stress. I would like to suggest a different approach. Stress will ebb and flow throughout the caregiver journey. So don't fight it; understand its uniqueness. This can help you find more effective ways to cope.

Why is caregiver stress so unique? First off, many different factors converge, including role confusion, problematic caregiving beliefs, ambiguous loss, and difficulty with saying no. This can thwart your ability to be mindful and to take care of yourself. Second, adult children caregivers often struggle with how to prioritize their own needs and the needs of their parents. This confounds their stress. Some caregivers focus so much on trying to meet the care recipient's needs that they lose sight of what their own needs are. It can then become difficult for them to recognize how stressed out they really are. This type of inner conflict can cause many caregivers to become depressed, burned-out, and—I believe—*dis-spirited*. "Dis-spirited" is a word I use to define disconnecting from your heart. And when you disconnect from your heart, you tend to cut yourself off from the people and activities that feed your spirit. When you become dis-spirited, you can feel out of balance and out of touch with your own needs.

Third, caregivers often have to care for someone who has a chronic illness, which has its own set of challenges. When your care recipient's condition continually changes, this can create ambiguity. And these changes are frequently unpredictable. In addition, the health of people with chronic illnesses often declines. These factors can make coping much more difficult. Recognizing the uniqueness of caregiver stress and *staying mindful* allows you to tackle these challenges by being focused, cautious, and aware.

Role Confusion and Role Changes

Two other issues can create immense stress for caregivers—role confusion and role change. *Role confusion* results from the changes that occur when an adult becomes ill or impaired, which in turn can confuse, blur, or dramatically alter your old roles. The following are some common statements from caregivers experiencing role confusion:

- "I feel like I am parenting my parent."
- "I sometimes don't feel like a wife anymore, but more like a nurse."
- "I love my mother, but her disease has changed our relationship so much."
- "I miss the father I knew before he became ill."
- "Having to be a caregiver has made me become a person I don't recognize."

- "I don't know if I am a we or an I."

Role confusion can place you in unfamiliar territory, which in turn can cause increased stress. To cope with role confusion, you have to shift your old role and accommodate to a new role. For adult children, this may require learning how to get more comfortable with your parent being more dependent on you. For spouses, role confusion requires the well spouse to shift into handling all the affairs of the couple, financial and personal. Well spouses feel like they sometimes have a spouse and sometimes don't.

Role change requires that you learn new ways to communicate and relate to one another. You also realize you can't share in the same way that you used to. You still can share, but you have to learn to expect that it won't be a reciprocal sharing. You may have to discover that the ways you spend time have to be different. For example, if you used to always talk over things together after you listened to music or watched a movie, you now may need to consider listening to music or watching movies together without sharing your thoughts afterward. Once you recognize and accept the changes, your confusion and stress will often lesson. You will be more capable of forging a new relationship with your care recipient. When you try to keep your roles the same or hope for things to remain unchanged, you can stress yourself out.

In the many years in which I counseled caregivers and led support groups, well spouses struggle the most with role confusion and role change. Well spouses have shared that at times they felt like a wife or husband and other times they felt like their spouse's caregiver. This aspect of caregiving can be quite stressful until the well spouse recognizes and accepts these role shifts. Explaining role confusion and role change has helped caregivers better understand why they felt the way they did. It also helped them accommodate to these changes. They recognized they had to let go of their old roles and begin to develop new roles. Ultimately they found more ease.

It takes a willingness to be compassionate and patient with yourself so that you can honor the emotions you are feeling. Ignoring or denying these role changes can increase stress and negatively affect your overall health and well-being.

Caregiver Ambiguous Loss

In addition to role confusion and role change, there is another unique issue that can cause a great deal of stress for caregivers—*ambiguous loss*. First described by Dr. Pauline Boss, ambiguous loss is a loss that is unclear, has no resolution, and no closure.[1] This concept can be particularly helpful in understanding the challenges of caring for someone with dementia. Ambiguous loss can become magnified as the care recipient's dementia constantly changes. Your care recipient may fluctuate between being absent and present. The person you are caring for may be only "partially available." This ambiguity, coupled with the loss of how you knew that person, can create tremendous strain. Because this type of loss is different for spousal caregivers than it is for adult children, I have created separate sections for each.

Ambiguous Loss for Spouses

As a spouse, ambiguous loss causes you to continually flip-flop between being the care recipient's spouse and then her caregiver. Flip-flopping between roles is confusing, awkward, and emotionally exhausting. In her book *Mainstay*, author Maggie Strong describes the struggle by noting that spousal caregivers can feel as if they are split between two worlds, the world of the sick and the world of the well.[2] In her case, she describes living in her husband's world, in which there were constant doctor appointments and his changing physical needs. And then she would have to shift into her own world, filled with personal and family obligations. She often couldn't predict what would happen each day or when a new health crisis would pop up. Essentially she was at her husband's beck and call. Through Maggie's experiences, she created a national organization called the Well Spouse Foundation,[3] which has support groups all over the country for people who are going through similar situations. You may want to check them out.

Ambiguous loss can also affect how and whether couples experience intimacy. For example, if your spouse has dementia, you may not be able to experience as much physical or emotional intimacy. This can be painful and sad for the caregiver and care recipient. Ambiguous loss and intimacy can be a particularly sensitive subject for spousal caregivers. This topic often came up in my support groups. Spousal caregivers appreciated having the opportunity to talk about this topic with other spouses. They mentioned they felt uncomfortable talking about intimacy with their friends or family and found that even their physicians rarely brought this topic up.

To help you understand ambiguous loss, I offer the following two examples of how spousal caregivers coped. I hope you can gather some ideas and strength from their experiences.

"Guilty or Not Guilty, That Is the Question"—Ambiguous Loss for a Spouse

I recall one support group meeting in which ambiguous loss was particularly evident. Jennifer had been married for more than thirty years and was caring for her husband, John, who had suffered a stroke ten years earlier. Jennifer was seventy-one years old and still full of life. She had recently met a gentleman in her church choir. Jennifer told the group how much she enjoyed Ross's company. She cherished singing with him, as well as their long talks after services. While Jennifer wasn't interested in being sexual with Ross, she admitted that she did miss male companionship. She struggled with her desire to see him socially and she felt guilty because she was still married. She shared with the group that at times she felt married and other times not. Yet John was still very much alive and she loved him dearly. She had no intentions of leaving him or not visiting with him. Jennifer didn't feel comfortable talking about this with any of her friends or family. But she felt people in this group would understand. After much discussion, the consensus was that she could still love her husband, be his advocate, *and* allow herself to enjoy Ross's companionship. Jennifer admitted to the group that she still felt guilty when she would spend time with Ross. However, the group helped Jennifer realize she could still love her husband and enjoy male companion friendship.

No doubt there are many issues and personal decisions that spousal caregivers have to make. Each person has to ultimately make a decision that is best for him or her. In my work with spousal caregivers, caregivers who were able to identify these role shifts were better able to cope with them. Here are some important points that can help all caregivers:

- Recognize the ambiguity of your situation.
- Realize it can feel like you are living in two different worlds.
- Acknowledge that your roles have changed.
- Honor all your feelings.
- Consider a support group where it will be safe to share uncomfortable feelings.

"When Love Is Not Enough"—Ambiguous Loss for a Spouse

A couple had come for counseling. Ted had Parkinson's disease and was still very interested in being sexual with his wife, Anne. Anne, on the other hand, felt more and more like Ted's caregiver. Because of how the disease impacted her husband physically, Anne found herself less sexually attracted to him. Ted was initially hurt by what Anne had shared. He had been in some denial about the changes his body was undergoing due to his Parkinson's disease. With some help from me, Ted eventually came to an understanding and felt less hurt by his wife. Anne made it very clear to him that she still loved him, but for her, their sexual relationship had changed. Ultimately, both of them had to find some new ways to be intimate with one another. They agreed they would find time for cuddling and make sure they hugged and kissed one another, at least in the morning and at bedtime.

Unfortunately, sexual intimacy can change when your care recipient has a chronic disease. It is important to try to find ways to accommodate your role change and the physical changes. Be willing to share your feelings honestly with one another. In some circumstances, however, these very intimate, personal choices can create tension between couples. If this is the case, then professional help may be needed to help you through this aspect of your journey together.

Ambiguous Loss for Adult Children

Adult children can also experience ambiguous loss. When your parent is no longer able to provide the advice or support you always relied upon, it can be upsetting. And when a parent loses some of his abilities or skills—such as being able to verbally communicate or take care of finances—adult children struggle with acknowledging that their roles have changed. This can be particularly painful when the adult child has to step in as the decision maker. It can result in feeling uncomfortable, guilt ridden, sad, resentful, and sometimes even angry. Taking on new responsibilities for a parent can cause some conflict for adult children. There are times when your parent may become angry with you or accuse you of trying to control him or take over. This can push your buttons big time. And you may begin to question whether you should be interfering or not. The following is an example of how an adult child handled this issue.

"Too Close for Comfort"—Ambiguous Loss for an Adult Daughter

Kate was struggling with her mother's dementia. Her mother, Maggie, was in the beginning stages of Alzheimer's disease. Maggie would have days when she was, as Kate would say, "with the program." Then there would be other days when Maggie was very confused and quite forgetful. Kate was torn between moving her mother to assisted living or keeping her at home. In many ways, she felt it was time to move Maggie. Just when she thought she was comfortable with her decision, her guilt would get the best of her and she would reverse her decision and state it would be best if her mother remained at home with caregiver help. With either scenario, Kate realized her mother would not be happy. Part of Kate's struggle was that she felt almost too close to her mother. Kate kept imagining what it would feel like to be in her mother's shoes. Plus, Kate's profound sadness in how her mother was changing was almost too painful for her to bear. She vacillated between wanting her mother to stay the same and knowing their roles were changing. Ambiguous situations such as this are quite common and can wreak havoc with caregivers' hearts and heads.

In our work together, I helped Kate get in touch with the ambiguity of her situation so she could recognize how the issues were creating problems. First, Kate had to acknowledge that her attachment to her mother was getting in the way of assessing Maggie's needs. Then, Kate had to realize that with Maggie's Alzheimer's disease, she would be prone to off and on days. Next, Kate would need to tackle the issue of where her mother should live. Even though Kate knew that Maggie would not want to move, she believed an assisted living community would be best. And last, but not least, Kate had to get past her guilt so she could make the best decision for her mother. She moved her mother and, for the most part, all went well.

Ambiguous situations are not easy to resolve. When caregivers can get in touch with how ambiguity affects caregiver stress, they have a better shot at coping with their situations. However, not every situation ends as successfully as Kate and Maggie's. This was the case with my next example.

"When Saying No Is Not Easy to Do" — Ambiguous Loss for a Son and His Father

James and Charles worked together in their family business. Charles owned a successful building supply company. After college, James came to work for his father, which thrilled Charles, as he hoped James would take over the company when he retired. However, Charles was a workaholic and derived most of his social interaction and self-esteem from being at work. He was also a bit controlling. Charles had Parkinson's disease and had difficulty with walking and balance. He was falling a lot, especially at work. James encouraged his father to retire because of the challenges posed by his disease. And, in truth, James was a bit embarrassed by his father's symptoms. Charles would hear none of that. He insisted on being at work every day so he could still be involved in the business. James was frustrated, not sure how to handle the situation, so he contacted me for a consultation. I met with James and found out that Charles would often fall asleep at his desk and was unable to grasp the business end of things. It appeared that he was also experiencing some dementia. A number of employees were making comments about his still being there. James noted that his father was completely unaware of how he came across at work.

In situations such as this, sometimes it's best for the adult child to move aside and let a professional intervene. I suggested that James take Charles to his neurologist and see if the neurologist would talk with him about retiring from work. The neurologist did talk with Charles, but it went in one ear and out the other. His father insisted upon continuing to work. When I inquired as to how Charles got to work, James said he arranged an employee to pick him up. It became clear that James was enabling his father by arranging transportation for his dad to get to work. While James understood he was enabling, he felt too guilty to tell his father he would not arrange transportation anymore. While it took some time, James benefited from some coaching and was able to take a stand with his father. Charles became very mad at him, which James was prepared for. The bottom line, not all family situations can be resolved without some tension and unease.

Understanding ambiguous loss and how it can interfere with coping is an important concept. Be mindful of how you might be trying to keep things the same. Doing so can result in more stress and unease. It can also cause feelings of guilt, a lack of setting limits, or avoiding decisions. Acknowledge the changes in your parent and allow yourself to process the feelings about those changes. In many ambiguous loss situations, there can be a positive outcome, but it takes perseverance and a willingness to sit with some discomfort.

CAREGIVER BELIEFS: BEING A MINDFUL CAREGIVER BEGINS WITH WHAT YOU THINK

> Everything begins with a thought.
> —Madeline Kay, *Living Serendipitously*, 107

Much of how we behave starts with how we think about things. As a caregiver, the way you think about your situation will influence how you cope. Mindfulness can be an effective way for you to get in touch with your beliefs and feelings. Becoming more aware of your beliefs helps clarify what those beliefs mean to you and how they can get in the way of self-care.

Becoming Aware of Your Entrenched Beliefs

Do any of these statements sound familiar?

- "No one can really take care of my husband as well as I can."
- "I know something bad will happen if I let someone else help out!"
- "There is no one who can really help me."
- "My husband won't let anyone else help."

I would imagine that to some of you these do sound familiar. And if they don't, I am certain that many of you have beliefs about how you "should" provide care. Let me define what I mean by beliefs. The word "belief" means holding a preconceived idea or expectation about something that is often based on cultural norms and values. In my experience, caregivers seem to have several similar beliefs about caregiving—many of which set them up for prolonged stress. I call these *entrenched* caregiver beliefs. Entrenched beliefs are beliefs that you hold onto very tightly and are uncomfortable to let go. Some of these beliefs are passed down from one generation to the next, and sometimes they are what you have become used to.

What is of upmost importance for caregivers is to recognize that trying to maintain some of these beliefs can cause great stress and discomfort. Furthermore, holding onto certain beliefs can unintentionally prevent you from recognizing that there may be others who could help out. The strong feelings and fears that are attached to these beliefs may make it scary and difficult to let go of them. Being mindful of your beliefs and the attached feelings can help you recognize what changes need to be made and how you can take better care of yourself. And that in itself is very empowering!

The following are some entrenched beliefs I have heard over the years. Let's examine them and see if you can identify with some of them. Then let's look at some of the barriers that can get in your way of letting them go.

No One Can Really Take Care of My Care Recipient as Well as I Can

> If we keep our eyes open long enough in the darkness, things will begin to take shape before us. We can learn things about ourselves that we never thought possible.
>
> —Naomi Levy, *To Begin Again*, 64

"No one can really take care of my care recipient as well as I can" is an entrenched belief that many caregivers tightly embrace. If you believe this, then ask yourself what feelings might be behind this belief. Are you afraid that your care recipient won't be taken care of as lovingly or caringly as you take care of him? Do you feel guilty that you should be caring for him? Are you worried that your care recipient might think you don't love him anymore? Or are you angry that family members put pressure on you to care for him? If you examine what's behind this belief, you can see feelings of *guilt, anger,* and *fear.* Those feelings can wear you down, hold you hostage, and stand in the way of your letting go of them

Using a mindfulness approach, sit quietly with each of the feelings. Become aware of your feelings and how they are linked to your beliefs. This can help you learn to accommodate to your situation more easily. Accommodating doesn't mean you have to entirely give up everything you believe. Instead, it means finding some wiggle room for new ways of thinking about caregiving so you can have new options available to you. It means reconsidering the definition of what it means to be a good caregiver. To do that, you have to let go of your list of "musts"—"I must . . . do whatever it takes, keep trying to make things right, place my care recipient ahead of myself." Interestingly, your "musts" don't usually involve taking care of yourself. Once you can surrender these "musts," you will begin to see things more realistically and be open to setting limits on what you can and can't do.

There Is Never Enough Time

> I felt like I was organizing the invasion of Normandy—so much to be
> handled, arranged, juggled, explained—to maintain his quality of life.
> —Olivia Hoblitzelle, *Ten Thousand Joys & Ten Thousand Sorrows*, 152

Truth be told, there is never enough time in our culture. And being a
caregiver only adds to this challenge. When I have asked caregivers why
they don't take better care of themselves, they share the following:

- "There isn't enough time to do all I need to do to take care of my
  parent and my family, let alone myself."
- "I don't have time to think about me, because I am constantly
  thinking and worrying about Dad."
- "It's my responsibility to give all my time to my husband."
- "I would feel guilty taking time for me. I don't want to be considered a selfish person."

Caregiving does take time. And more often than not, it can take a lot
of time! As the title of the best-selling book on Alzheimer's care, *The 36-
Hour Day*,[4] suggests, caring for someone with a chronic illness is like
living a thirty-six-hour day! Or as one caregiver said, "I feel like my
mother's illness sucks the life out of me and I can't find the time or the
energy to replenish myself."

Holding onto entrenched beliefs about "not enough time" can sabo-
tage you. For example, many of you may believe *you have to handle every
aspect* of caregiving. When you believe that you have to handle everything, it absolutely sets you up for having no time for yourself. I can't
begin to tell you how many overwhelmed and exhausted caregivers
would say to me: "No one else would step up to the plate," "I am the only
one who can take care of my mother," or "Everyone else is so busy." At
face value, these statements might be true. However, it's important to
examine those beliefs carefully and consider there may be other options.

The following are some questions to consider. Recognize that in order
for you to find some time for yourself, you will have to *change the way you
answer* each of these questions.

- Do you believe it is *your* responsibility to be the primary caregiver?
  If so, why?
- Have you *asked for help*, and if not, why not? Are you afraid of being
  turned down?
- Are you so worn out you can barely navigate?
- Do you make assumptions about who might be available to help
  before you check it out?
- Do you assume that family members or others will not help?
- Does your *guilt* stand in your way?

- Do you believe that others will think badly of you if you ask for help?

If you said "yes" to even one of these questions, I suspect you are already struggling with taking time for yourself. So what needs to change so you can begin to let go? I suggest you consider a mindfulness approach. Quiet your thoughts so you can pay attention with purpose. Then you will be more able to connect to your heart in order to get in touch with how you feel. When you do so, you are more apt to let go of your entrenched beliefs. First, acknowledge that you are holding onto an entrenched belief; examine the feelings around that belief and how those feelings serve as a barrier to finding time for self-care. Next, make a commitment to ease up on that belief so you can make room for yourself. This does not have to be an all-or-nothing solution. If you can't or won't let go, you will most likely end up on a course for caregiver burnout and caregiver numb-out. Just as cars can't run on fumes, neither can caregivers.

Another positive aspect of applying mindfulness is that the approach requires you to stay more focused in the present moment. And if you stay more focused in the present moment, you can't drag in a past belief. Author Ram Dass offers a very interesting perspective in this regard. He states that "in the present moment there is no time."[5] This is an important concept for caregivers. If you are constantly worrying about what you have to do next, you are not staying in the present. Instead, you are using your time worrying, which only exacerbates the situation. In essence, you create a vicious cycle of continually feeling like you don't have enough time. Think about a moment in which you were so absorbed in a movie, a piece of music, or a story. You lost track of time. Your mind was not involved, only your heart. When caregivers get caught up in their heads and drag the future or past into the present, then they end up focusing on what they lack. When you apply mindfulness to caregiving, you stay more in the present so that each experience is just that, an experience. This is especially important because your care recipient's situation can change from moment to moment. And every new moment is an opportunity for a different experience.

"I Have to Make the Right Decision"

> Always do your best, no more and no less.
> —Don Miguel Ruiz, *The Four Agreements*, 75

Another entrenched belief that can cause tremendous stress is when you believe you *have* to make the *right* decision or something very wrong will happen. In the above quote, the word "best" is used instead of the word "right." Let me explain why this substitution of words can make a huge difference for caregivers. Throughout our lives, there has been a great emphasis on making sure things are done "the *right* way." I remember my father saying to me, "Nancy, if you can't do it right, don't do it at all!" In my work with caregivers, I have found that trying to get to *right* often makes things difficult. Trying to make the *right decision* can immobilize caregivers. For example, you may be afraid of making the wrong decision or you may feel so worried about making the right decision that you make no decision at all. This can leave you feeling stuck, overwhelmed, and plain old frustrated. You can get caught up in believing you must do what others think is *right* or what your care recipient thinks is *right*. Embracing "best" can transform the caregiver experience. It can be the difference between walking alongside stress, instead of stress walking all over you!

Ruiz's quote fits beautifully for caregivers. Essentially by doing your best, no more and no less, you don't have to come up with the perfect solution or the absolute right choice. He chooses the word "best" because it is much more forgiving and there is room for opportunity and compromise. *Best* allows you to examine all your options and choose what ultimately appears to be the optimum for all involved. So as a mindful caregiver, consider doing what is best, so you can move beyond "right." Taking this approach will help you work toward the "best" possible solution or decision.

The statements below offer some new perspectives on choosing best. Best:

- Frees you from not getting stuck in "right."
- Provides the opportunity to examine all your options.
- Helps pave a path for decisions to be made more easily.
- Helps you set limits.

The following example describes a granddaughter who was stuck in one of her entrenched beliefs, "having to make the right decision," and how she was able to get to the "best decision" for her grandmother.

"When Right Is Not Always Best"—Granddaughter Emily

Emily invited her eighty-nine-year-old grandmother, Sally, who lived out of state, to come visit her for the Easter holiday. During her stay, Sally fell and broke her hip. She ended up requiring surgery and then rehabilitative care. Although Sally recovered fairly well, the rehab staff strongly felt that Sally needed more care. The staff told both Emily and Sally that it was not safe for Sally to go home to her own apartment, especially without caregiver help. They recommended that Sally go into an assisted living facility for at least a month or two. The rehab professionals felt that Sally required careful supervision and a watchful eye.

At the hospital discharge meeting, Sally was adamant that she would go nowhere else but back to her old apartment. Emily was beside herself.

She felt caught between doing what the rehab professionals said was safest for her grandmother and, at the same time, wanting to be respectful of Sally's wishes. She was struggling with how to make the *right* decision for Sally. Recognizing how upset Emily and Sally were, the rehab social worker referred Emily to me. I met with Emily and Sally and quickly realized each of them believed they knew what the "right decision" was. Sally felt the right decision was for her to go home and get additional physical therapy there. She felt that if she needed help, she could ask one of her neighbors. On the other hand, Emily felt the right decision was for Sally to move into an assisted living place near her. Both were equally attached to their respective decisions. It was causing immense stress between the two, despite the fact that they had always been close.

I proposed that they work toward a different type of decision. Instead of staying attached to what they thought was *right*, I asked them to consider what might be *best*. Working toward best encouraged them to consider all options and provided an opening for compromise. They set up another meeting, which resulted in a solution that gave each some satisfaction. Emily's grandmother did move back home but agreed to daily help from a professional caregiver for the first few weeks of her return. Sally also agreed to wear a lifeline pendant. Emily committed to visiting her grandmother once a quarter to see how things were progressing. While neither was completely satisfied, they at least felt that the "best decision" for that time had been made.

Hopefully, this section helps illustrates how some beliefs can interfere with being able to make effective decisions. The next section looks at what you say to yourself and how that influences coping and self-care.

BEING MINDFUL OF WHAT YOU SAY TO YOURSELF: COMPASSIONATE SELF-CARE

This next concept is one I hope caregivers will welcome with open arms, learning to be compassionate with yourself. *Compassionate self-care* asks that you pay attention to what you say to yourself about how you provide care. How you talk to yourself can directly affect how you feel, the decisions you make, and how you provide care.

For example, if you tell yourself . . .

- "My situation is impossible and will never get better."
- "Someday I will take better care of myself, but I just don't have the time now."
- "I don't have the time to focus on me. I have to focus on him."
- "I can't let anyone else take care of my mother."

Then, most likely what you say and believe becomes your truth.

However, if you tell yourself . . .

- "My situation can change, and I have to be open for whatever comes my way."
- "I will make the time to take care of myself, which will make me a kinder, more patient caregiver to my husband."
- "I do have the time to focus on me, because I matter."
- "Letting others help care for my mother not only gives me some respite but also adds new people and meaning into my mother's life."

Then, most likely *you will* be more able to cope and find positive solutions. So remember, only *you* have control over what you say to yourself.

Author Madeleine Kay believes the words you say to yourself and others can influence your behavior.[6] In the chart below, she demonstrates the power of words. Consider how each of the columns of words can either *discourage* or *support* change.

Eliminate This Word	Replace it with This Word
Can't	Can
If	When
Why?	Why not?
Limited	Unlimited
Should	Could
Impossible	Possible
Wish	Will
Someday	Now

Now let's apply this to caregiving.

Let's first start with the set of words in the *Eliminate* column. These words tend to be negative and can serve as major roadblocks to change and moving forward. They also tend to place blame and shame on the caregiver. These words reinforce the feeling that your situation is hopeless and that change is impossible. The words in the *Replace* column tend to be positive and can open doors and provide new pathways. They give you hope and a sense that change is possible. When providing care, focus on the words in the *Replace* column. Hopefully, this will decrease your stress and help you feel more comfortable and confident in your ability to handle whatever comes your way. And if these words don't quite fit for you, substitute the words in each column with your own.

COMPASSIONATE SELF-CARE MESSAGES

Once you are more aware of what you say to yourself, you then have to take steps to give yourself *positive self-care messages*. All caregivers need their own set of positive self-care messages. I will jump-start you with some positive self-care messages to consider and hope you will also add some of your own:

- I will stay open to change.
- I will learn to be with the unknown.
- I will allow myself to feel the fear and still move forward.
- I am the one that has to accommodate to the changes, not my care recipient.
- I can accept the help of others.
- I will take time for me, because I matter.
- I will do my best.

Take time each morning and night to sit with these compassionate self-care messages and allow them to flow to your heart. Compassionate self-care requires being mindful of what beliefs you hold, both positive and negative. Once acknowledged, you can begin to slowly let go of the negative beliefs that keep you trapped. You can begin to replace them with positive beliefs that allow you to take care of yourself and provide the best care to your care recipient.

Letting go of some of your entrenched beliefs, being more mindful of what you say to yourself, and committing to giving yourself positive self-care messages can certainly pave the way for finding more time for you. However, there is still one more hurdle you have to get over: learning to set limits and get to a positive no.

Learning to Set Limits

Setting limits means learning when to say no. And it's not easy. Setting limits requires that you become aware of what you realistically can and can't do. Doing so can cause disappointment, but it is essential for self-care. So start with a limit that you believe you most likely *will be able* to accomplish. For example, think about a friend or family member who might be okay with you setting a limit. Talk to her and clearly communicate your needs. Perhaps it is a statement that you can't do it all and need their help. Perhaps it's saying no to their request. Experiencing success helps pave the way for trying other options. And most importantly, it reinforces that you matter too!

Setting limits takes practice. The first time or two that you set a limit, you may feel guilty. Feeling guilty is a part of feeling concerned. Let yourself feel some of the guilt, as it is normal and to be expected. Over time, the feelings will lessen. Below are some ideas of how to set limits:

- I am important and I matter, so I just can't do this right now.
- I care about you and me, so I need to do this for both of us.
- Let me think about it and give you my answer later (sometimes you may need time in order to say no).
- I know you will be disappointed with my answer, and I am sorry . . . . I am going to do this for me.

Setting limits requires considering your needs as well as your care recipients. You have to be a part of the equation together with your care recipient. Setting limits is not only healthy for you to do but also reinforces that you matter. When you don't set limits, you often end up *overfunctioning*.

Overfunctioning is when *you* believe you must take on all the responsibility. Overfunctioning people tend to be labeled as reliable or having their "act together." When you overfunction, people who could possibly help out will often underfunction. Underfunctioning people count on you taking charge. In her book *The Dance of Anger*, Harriet Lerner suggests that many interactions tend to be overfunctioning/underfunctioning "dances" between two people.[7] Usually there is one caregiver in the family who tends to be the overfunctioning adult and one or more underfunctioning adults. Overfunctioning and underfunctioning adults reinforce each other's behaviors. And this can result in emotionally intense and blaming behavior. In my practice, I find that many caregivers are not aware of how much they tend to overfunction. They hold tight to the belief that no one else will help out. Although this is no doubt true in certain situations, when asked for help and support, most people will rise to the occasion.

Let me provide a typical caregiver example. Joan was taking care of her husband, John. She felt like she had to do it all: care for him, keep the house up, do all the shopping, cook all the meals, and still on occasion babysit for her grandchildren. While Joan enjoyed doing some of these things, she also resented doing some tasks. Joan is a prime example of an overfunctioning person. And her overfunctioning and not setting limits created much internal turmoil for her. In order to stop overfunctioning, Joan had to be willing to do the following:

- Step back and separate out which tasks she enjoyed doing and which ones she didn't enjoy doing.
- Then she had to clarify how much time each task took and which of those she enjoyed and which she didn't. As difficult as it might be, sometimes caregivers have to put limits on even the enjoyable tasks.
- Next, she had to recognize and prioritize which personal and family tasks she could let go of. For example, perhaps she would have to let go of her belief that her home had to be kept perfectly and let other family members do some of the grocery shopping or cooking.

- She had to be willing to delegate some of these tasks to others. This meant being willing to ask others for help.
- And lastly, she had to acknowledge her guilt, learn to say no, and then let it go.

Mustering up courage, Joan learned to not worry so much. She learned to be okay if the house wasn't perfect. She ordered meals out and even froze meals for later. She asked her sister-in-laws to help with the grocery shopping, and let her daughter know that she wouldn't always be able to babysit the grandkids.

Getting to a Positive No

> Whether and how we say No determines the very quality of our lives. It is perhaps the most important word for us to learn to say gracefully and effectively.
> —William Ury, *The Power of a Positive No*, 5

Early on in our lives, as children, we were introduced to the word "no." At times, our parents used the word loudly and firmly. And most of the time, we listened. It was a word that we respected. Yet, as adults, saying no can feel almost impossible, especially in caregiving situations. Saying no can feel harsh, especially to caregivers who pride themselves on being kind, loving, and supportive. Plus, saying no has different meanings and can be heard positively or negatively by different people. For some, caregivers believe that no means they have been unsuccessful as caregivers or are inadequate. For others, it just means they are tired or need a change. It can also serve as *just a pause*, a breathing period, or a time to explore other options. *No* is one of the best ways to establish healthy boundaries. And boundaries help caregivers distinguish between their own needs and the needs of the care recipient.

Author William Ury shares, "*No* is the tension between exercising your power and tending to your relationship."[8] He implies that people can misuse the word, either by accommodating people by saying yes, when they really mean no, or by attacking and saying the word *no* with harshness. And lastly, we may try to avoid the situation or person by saying nothing at all.

There are many reasons you may have difficulty saying no.

- You may be concerned that by saying no you won't be able to stick to your conviction.
- You get caught between *how to say no* and *when to say no*.
- For many, saying no is more difficult because you know there will be consequences for saying no.
- Saying no can sometimes create self-doubt and anxiety.

Caregivers have all sorts of excuses for not saying no.

- "I can't say no, I don't want to hurt their feelings."
- "How can I say no, when I know I am supposed to say yes?"
- "Will I regret saying no and how will it come back to haunt me?"
- "What will others think of me if I say no?"

So How Can Caregivers Get to a Positive No?

> A "No" uttered from deepest conviction is better and greater than a "Yes" uttered to please, or what is worse, to avoid trouble.
> —Mahatma Gandhi, cited by William Ury, *The Power of a Positive No*, 7

First, you have to acknowledge you don't have to do everything. You have to remember that everyone has different thresholds for coping with stress. It's important to know your threshold and be able to admit that you need help. Second, you need to learn not to say yes when you mean no. This is when a mindfulness approach can really help. Remember, *pause and take a deep breath*. Then tell the person you would like to think about it first. This allows you to step back and get in touch with what you need to do to take care of yourself. It's important to remember that saying yes when you really mean no can encourage resentment and anger.

The best example of how to get to a positive no comes from Pam, who was trying to support her parents. Pam's mother was becoming more and more exhausted and frustrated caring for her father. Her mother was also relying more and more on Pam to help out. Her mother would call Pam and ask her to come over after work and stay with her father while she ran errands. Over time, these requests increased and Pam was feeling resentful and even angry. She dreaded the phone calls from her mom and struggled with how to say no. Pam had been contemplating asking her mother to consider hiring a part-time home care aide. Yet she couldn't find the courage to bring it up without feeling guilty and ashamed.

I suggested to Pam that there may be some ways to say no in a more positive way. We first talked through all the situations in which she felt resentful and angry. Next, we discussed what Pam was willing and able to do to help. Then, we identified additional ways her mother could get some support, such as from people at their church, various day programs for her father, and possibly a professional caregiver to come over for a few hours a week. Pam spoke with her mother and, to her surprise, found out that her mother was actually unaware of her daughter's feelings and was quite willing to consider other options. Relieved, the tension was broken and the two were able to regain their close and supportive relationship.

A note of caution: Not all situations turn out this positively. There will be times when the parent or other caregiving adult will not be open and willing. In such cases, it might be best to have a professional intervene. Getting to a "positive no" takes being proactive, recognizing what you can and cannot do, and carefully thinking through all your options. The results—taking care of yourself—are certainly worth the effort and the only way toward healthy self-care.

Part of limit setting may also involve letting go of some of your responsibilities and getting others to help out. Here are some ideas for that.

- Build a support network of people who can be "friendly visitors" to your care recipient, letting them know they are an important part of your support team.
- Think of tasks or errands you do on a regular basis and see if you can either hire someone to help or get a volunteer from your place of worship or other organization.
- Give yourself a break from visiting your parent or care recipient by asking one of your friends to pinch-hit for you. Consider a day program that can give you some respite and provide your care recipient with socialization and structure.
- Ask a family member to stay with your care recipient so you can have a night out.

Beginning to let others help you when you aren't in a crisis provides you with the courage to ask for help over more challenging situations or issues.

A lot has been covered in this chapter. I want to insist that you have to be your own best self-care advocate. You have to give yourself permission to invest in a self-care plan. As your journey unfolds, you may want to go back and review some of the sections. Remember, learning something new takes practice and patience. In closing, I offer you the *Caregiver Bill of Rights.*[9] I hope you will find a prominent place to post this in your house. And I hope it helps remind you of the importance of self-care.

CAREGIVER BILL OF RIGHTS

I have the right to take care of myself. This is not an act of selfishness. It will give me the ability to take better care of my loved one.

I have the right to seek help from others even though my loved one may object. I know the limits of my own endurance and strength.

I have the right to maintain parts of my own life that do not include the person I care for, just as I would if he were healthy. I know that I do everything that I reasonably can do for this person. I have the right to do some things just for myself.

I have the right to get angry, be depressed, and express difficult feelings once in a while.

I have the right to reject any attempt by my loved one to make me do things out of guilt or anger. (It doesn't matter if she knows that she is doing it or not.)

I have the right to get consideration, affection, forgiveness, and acceptance for what I do for my loved one, as I offer these in return.

I have the right to take pride in what I'm doing. And I have the right to applaud the courage it has taken to meet the needs of my loved one.

I have the right to protect my individuality. I also have the right to a life that will sustain me in times when my loved one no longer needs my full-time help.

—Author Unknown

NOTES

1. Pauline Boss, *Loving Someone Who Has Dementia* (San Francisco: Jossey-Bass, 2011).

2. Maggie Strong, *Mainstay* (Cambridge, Mass.: Bradford Books, 1997).

3. Well Spouse Foundation, "Well Spouse Foundation," www.wellspouse.org.

4. Nancy L. Mace and Peter V. Rabins, *The 36-Hour Day* (New York: Warner Books, 1999).

5. Ram Dass, *Still Here: Embracing Aging, Changing, and Dying* (New York: Riverhead Books, 2000), 135.

6. Madeleine Kay, *Living Serendipitously: Keeping the Wonder Alive* (Flat Rock: Chrysalis, 2003), 54.

7. Harriet Lerner, *The Dance of Anger: A Woman's Guide to Changing the Patterns of Intimate Relationships* (New York: HarperCollins, 2005).

8. William Ury, *The Power of a Positive No: Save the Deal, Save the Relationship, and Still Say No* (New York: Bantam Dell, 2007), 10.

9. The National Cancer Institute at the National institutes of Health, "When Someone You Love Is Being Treated for Cancer," www.cancer.gov.cancertopics/coping/when-someone-you-love-is-treated.

FOUR

Incorporating Mindfulness into Self-Care

Creative Ideas and Exercises

In the beginner's mind there are many possibilities, but in the expert's there are few.

—Shunryu Suzuki Roshi, *Zen Mind, Beginner's Mind*

NEW WAYS TO CONSIDER TAKING CARE OF YOURSELF

To encourage you to think differently about self-care, I ask you to consider using what the Buddhists call a *beginner's mind*. A beginner's mind requires treating everything as a new experience and being willing to open yourself to new ideas with no judgments or expectations. Caregivers need a variety of ways to take care of themselves. This chapter provides many tips and suggestions that hopefully will be helpful to you.

Let's get started by looking at a few questions for you to ponder before we dive into specific techniques.

Your Needs vs. Others' Needs

- Do you consider the needs of others?
- Do you place everyone's needs before your own?
- Do you balance others' needs with your own?

These questions are important because they help you become more conscious of whether you tune into what you need or whether you are mainly focused on what your care recipient and others need from you. In my practice with caregivers, I have noticed that caregivers place their own needs last. In fact, some caregivers feel that if they pay attention to their needs they are being selfish.

Rest

- What does it mean to truly rest?
- Why is it important?
- How does it replenish your spirit?

Whenever I mention rest, caregivers look at me as if I am speaking a foreign language. How can they rest when there is so much to be done and not enough time to do it all? Believe it or not, there are many different ways to incorporate rest into your daily routine, and it can take as little as five or ten minutes each day. Later in this chapter, I provide some suggestions. And, of course, true rest means making sure you get a good night's sleep or that you take a nap during the day. Research demonstrates that a good night's sleep and short daily naps are effective ways to combat stress and replenish yourself.[1]

Comforting Yourself

How do you comfort yourself? There are positive and negative ways of feeling comfort.

Positive comforts might involve:

- Gardening or sitting in a garden.
- Finding an exercise routine that makes you feel good.
- Hanging out with friends.
- Finding a peaceful space to pray or just be quiet.

Negative comforts might include:

- Indulging in too much food or alcohol or addictive behaviors that distract and affect you adversely.
- Keeping yourself so busy you have no time to feel tired, depressed, or stressed.

Do you refuse comfort? If so, why?

- Those of you who can relate to this question may find that guilt can get in your way or that you may feel selfish about allowing yourself to feel comfortable.

Becoming more mindful of how you comfort yourself is critical to self-care. While it's wonderful to receive comfort from others, caregivers also have to learn how to self-soothe.

Balance Your Head and Heart

- How do you move away from your head and into your heart?
- How do you get rid of the mental chatter that keeps you blocked from your heart?

Mental chatter refers to all those thoughts that can run around in your head. Your mind is stuck on overdrive. You might spend a lot of time thinking and worrying about things that might happen or get trapped in "what if" thinking. Mental chatter interferes with paying attention to your heart and intuition. Moving away from your head and into your heart requires that you stop and quiet your mind so you can connect to your heart. Mindfulness teaches you how to quiet these thoughts, so you can put a stop to the mental chatter.

Surrender to What Is

- What does the word "surrender" mean to you?
- Do you believe that surrender can encourage strength and ease?
- Or do you think that surrendering means giving up?

Many people believe that surrendering is giving up. As you read further in this chapter, you will learn ways to surrender that don't mean giving up—but instead, letting go.

Some of you may be familiar with the Serenity Prayer. I would like to offer this as a way to think about surrendering. For those of you not comfortable with using the term *God*, you can either leave it out or substitute the word that feels best for you.

Serenity Prayer

God grant me the serenity to accept the things I cannot change; courage to change the things I can; and wisdom to know the difference.

—Reinhold Niebuhr, cited in John Bartlett, *Bartlett's Familiar Quotations*, 735

Fun

- Do you still make time to have some fun in your life?
- What do you consider to be fun?
- Has your idea of fun changed? If so, how?

When I pose this question to caregivers, they often look stunned. Yet finding time for fun and laughter is essential to keeping balance and finding ease during the caregiving journey.

I hope that being more conscious about these questions and the way you answered them will help you become more aware of what you need to do to begin to take care of you!

SELFISH/SELFLESS/SELF-FULL

There is a fine line between dedication and martyrdom, between self-lessness and self-preservation.
—Claire Berman, *Caring for Yourself while Caring for Your Aging Parents*,
171

For the longest time, even though I visited my mother at her nursing home once or twice during the week, I believed that I *had to visit* my mother each weekend. I knew that weekends tended to have fewer programs and activities. And staffing changes were more frequent, which meant that the staff was not as familiar with my mother. Furthermore, visiting on the weekends allowed me more time to spend with her.

Ten years into my caregiving journey with my mom, I became angry about having to visit every weekend. I resented having to build my weekends around my mother. However, thinking about not visiting caused incredible waves of guilt to wash over me. I battled with thinking, "She is my mother, and I *should* visit her on the weekend no matter what." I just couldn't seem to make peace with this issue. I had begun to dread the weekends. I would only give myself permission to not visit her on the weekend when I was either out of town or sick. It was disheartening and distressing to admit the beliefs I held about visiting were causing me so much stress and resistance to changing how often I visited. Reading this you might think I was rather *selfish* or not a very caring daughter. You may wonder how I could be resentful of visiting her when I was only doing so a couple times a week. Or maybe you're thinking that it shouldn't bother me since I didn't care for her round-the-clock.

Yet each caregiver situation is unique, with many layers of relational history. Being able to honor the uniqueness of your journey is the first step toward acknowledging your resistance, so you can move forward. In coming to terms with my resistance, I realized that some of my resistance stemmed from emotional baggage from former years with my mother. I had been caring for her on and off since I was thirteen years old, as she had a bipolar disease. I decided to apply a mindfulness approach and stop judging myself and worrying about what others would think of me. I loved my mother very much and knew I would always make sure she was well cared for.

It was during my struggles with how to carve out quality time and visits with my mother that I began to think about the words *selfish*, *selfless*, and a new word I created, *self-full*. Let me define each of the words. I define *selfish* as individuals who do not consider the needs of others. And at times, selfish individuals can hurt other people's feelings in order to make sure their needs get met.

At times, I felt *selfless*. Selfless individuals are people who place everyone's needs before their own, often at their own expense. Selfless people tend to push their needs aside for others, even if they are becoming depressed and drained. I wanted to take better care of myself, so I wasn't caught between feeling stressed out, angry, and then guilty. I also realized that kind of energy was not healthy for my mother or me. I wanted to become *self-full*. I define *self-full* as being respectfully and thoughtfully aware of others but not at the expense of yourself. It requires being able to set personal limits and boundaries and knowing when to advocate for yourself.

I became self-full by finally letting go of my beliefs about having to visit every weekend, as well as my concern about how others would think of me. While it was not easy putting those beliefs aside, I realized there were other options—I could ask friends to visit, I could call my mother, I could send her a card. Or I could just "be" with my choice and know it was okay. I share this example in the hope that you will consider how you can be self-full.

You may find that some of my ways of being self-full might fit for you. If not, remember that being self-full requires staying aware of all your options and being open to letting others help. There are professionals from which you can get support and lots of online resources listed in appendix B. I encourage you to check them out.

SELF-CARE: CREATIVE IDEAS AND EXERCISES

Before healing others, heal thyself.
—Nigeria, *A Tiny Treasure of African Proverbs*

Applying mindfulness to self-care requires a willingness to be aware of how you are feeling so that you take care of yourself in an intentional way. Throughout your caregiving journey, you will need different ways to take care of yourself that work for you at that given moment. Remember to be patient and compassionate with yourself. That is how you become a mindful caregiver.

Learning to Pause

You may wonder what pausing has to do with self-care. Pausing means that you stop for a moment, take a deep breath, and slow yourself down before you say or do something you then regret. You stop "doing" and analyze your situation and what you are experiencing. For example, are you tired, inpatient, frustrated, or fearful? These feelings can wreak havoc with your heart and spirit and cause you to *react* or *act out*. Pausing disrupts habitual behaviors and opens up the possibility for new and creative ways of coping. Pausing gives you the opportunity to make better choices because you look at your situation from all different angles. It affords the opportunity to "try on" what you are thinking before you start doing.

Rest and Sleep

Rest and sleep are essential to good self-care. Lack thereof can be detrimental to your health, as well as the health of your care recipient. It is well documented that rest and sleep are the mainstays to health and wellness, as rest can give you a completely different perspective of your situation. Rest allows you to:

- Heal
- Reflect
- Give thanks and receive blessings
- Be more patient and compassionate
- Face whatever may lie ahead with a renewed sense of calm
- Appreciate the special moments

Rest and sleep replenish not just the body but the mind and the spirit as well. Yet caregivers often report that they don't rest during the day and sleep as little as four or five hours a night.

Most caregivers share that it's hard to get a good rest at night either because they are always listening for whether the care recipient is getting up, or they get awakened during the night. There is no easy answer, but there are some things you might want to consider. In general, many of us are so conditioned to keep going, to move faster or do more. Rest feels not only a waste of time, but it also means we are not "doing enough." My hope is that you will consider looking at the importance of rest in a different way after reading this section. Most people need at least six solid hours of sleep—eight hours is even better. In addition, I would encourage you to build some *true rest* into your day. True rest is when you stop what you are doing and find a way to quiet yourself, especially your mind. The important thing about true rest is that it can easily be built into your day and isn't time consuming. Even five to ten minutes of rest several times a day can be quite rejuvenating.

The following are examples of how to incorporate five minutes of rest into your daily routine.

- Seek out a quiet space to take deep breaths and quiet your mind
- Find a phrase that helps you, such as "I'm resting and restoring my body, mind, and spirit" or "I replenish myself with each and every breath"
- Relax your body with some stretching

- Go outside and garden. Prune, pull weeds, water flowers . . .
- Sing
- Walk outside and breathe in the beauty around you
- Listen to some soothing music
- Call a friend
- Watch something funny on television or the web

All of these examples are ways to help you decompress and regenerate. *True rest* doesn't require time as much as it requires a willingness to stop your constant doing and busyness. It requires a mindfulness approach, paying attention to what you need so your spirit and soul can be nourished.

Another powerful way to obtain rest is through exercises that teach you how to quiet your mind so you can connect back to your heart. I hope the following information and exercises will help. They are simple, easy ways for you to rest and take better care of yourself.

Meditation

Meditation teaches you to quiet your mind and body so your whole being can be at rest. It helps you connect to your body by listening to your breathing and heartbeat. It helps slow you down and calm your spirit.

Benefits of Meditation

- It brings you into a deeper awareness, so you can become more self-aware.
- It helps you to physically learn to relax.
- It helps you stay in the present moment.
- It can help calm you, particularly when you are anxious or stressed.
- Spiritually, it can help to reenergize.

Ways You Can Approach Meditation

There are many different kinds of meditation practices and techniques. I suggest that you meditate in a way that feels most comfortable for you. You don't have to sit in a particular position or pose or be in a specific setting. Meditation can be practiced at home, at work, in your garden, or even in your car!

Traditional Meditation Practices and Approaches

There are many different traditional meditation practices that may be familiar to you. Some common examples include:

- Mindfulness-based stress reduction

- Buddhist practices
- Zen practices

There are various classes you can take to learn how to meditate. You can also find all sorts of books, CDs, or YouTube videos that can teach you the different traditional meditation practices.

Nontraditional Meditation Approaches

For some of you who may be a bit timid about considering meditation or those of you who have tried more traditional approaches and were unsuccessful, there is hope. Two important elements are needed: You must be willing to carve out some time and then commit to practicing whatever way you choose to meditate.

Let me help you get started. First off, you have to give yourself permission to take a break. You deserve it, and the one you are caring for likely wants you to have a break. It is good for you both. To begin with, take a five-minute break. Then try increasing the number of five-minute breaks you take each day. Once you establish a practice of taking a break, you can become more aware of how important it is to slow down. Next, think of an activity that calms and relaxes you, especially those that help you temporarily forget about your worries and stresses. Write them down and keep that list handy. Now you are ready to attempt to incorporate meditation into self-care.

The following are some examples of ways that are comforting and very meditative for me:

- Gardening—I have always felt relaxed when gardening. I can play in the dirt and forget the world.
- Photographing flowers—For me, there is nothing better than sitting with a beautiful flower and photographing all of its splendor.

Both of these activities release my mind from my worry and stress. Some of my clients have shared ways they have found to be meditative, such as walking, running, swimming, or hiking. These activities are active. In contrast, other clients prefer reading, singing, or yoga, which are more passive. Think about what brings you peace and relaxation; maybe it's cooking a healthy meal with soft music playing in the background, enjoying a glass of wine on your patio, or browsing the sales racks at your favorite department store. Whatever it is, identify it, and make time for it.

What's most important is that you find a way to shut off what the Buddhists call your "monkey mind." Monkey mind is the mental chatter that feeds your stress. Being able to release your worries and stress, even if it's for a short period of time, is energizing in a positive way. I share this with you because I strongly believe in meditation. It is a wonderful way to clear and quiet the mind, rest your heart, and nourish your spirit.

A Meditation for Caregivers

When researching information about meditation, I came across the *Loving Kindness Meditation*, which has become a great source of calm and strength to me and to others. It was written by Jack Kornfield and can be found in his book *A Path with a Heart*.[2] I believe this meditation can be particularly soothing for caregivers. To use this meditation, please find a quiet and comfortable space, and then softly say to yourself:

> May I be filled with loving-kindness
> May I be safe from inner and outer dangers
> May I be well in body and mind
> May I be at ease and happy

I have shared this meditation with many caregivers who now say they either begin or end their day with this meditation.

Breathing and Breath

We all tend to take our breathing for granted, that is, until we get a powerful reminder from getting the wind knocked out, choking on something, or even being under water too long. These situations can be quite frightening and cause panic when you realize you can't breathe. A more dramatic way to think about breathing is to realize that a single breath can be the barrier between life and death. What we often fail to recognize is how powerfully healing our breath and breathing can be to calming and healing us.

Paying attention to your breathing, particularly when you are stressed or emotionally upset, can help you remain calm, grounded, and empowered. If you can learn to pay attention to your breathing, some of your stress and anxiety can be alleviated. Breathing can help you remain calmer and may even lower your blood pressure.

The Importance of a Breathing Exercise

Building a breathing exercise into your day is quite simple. It requires that you move away from your care recipient and find a peaceful, quiet, and comfortable spot. If possible, sit as straight as you can, take a deep breath in through your nose, and breathe out through your mouth. Try to make sure that when you breathe in and out, your tummy moves. Spending just five to ten minutes of focused breathing a few times a day can help you remain a bit calmer.

Ideas for Breathing Exercises

There are many different approaches to help you calm your mind so you can focus on your breath. The following are some ideas to consider as you prepare for your breathing exercise.

- Turn the lights out, close your eyes, and sit quietly.
- Use a meditation bell or chime to help you focus and prepare to quiet yourself.
- Turn on comforting, quiet music.
- Place your hand on your heart to calm yourself.
- Step outside to breathe in the outside air.

Breathing Meditation

There are many different meditations you can find to help you. Below is a simple breathing meditation that I have created for caregivers. Find a quiet place, consider placing your hand over your heart, feel your heartbeat, and think about breathing out all the worries of the day. Quietly say the following as you breathe in and out:

> I take in compassion and exhale fear
> I take in kindness and exhale anger
> I take in joy and exhale sadness
> I take in ease and exhale discomfort.

This is just one example of a breathing meditation. You certainly can consider making up your own. What's most critical is remembering the importance of intentional breathing. Try to practice it a couple of times a day.

Prayer

Prayer is another way to calm the mind and connect to your heart. Prayer can help you find strength and center yourself. For some, prayer is the best way to get close to God. For others, it is a way to communicate with your soul. It helps you to "keep the faith" and garner courage and strength. Prayer can be expressed in music and movement. You don't need words in order to pray, and you don't have to be religious. You just have to be willing to reach out beyond yourself. I highly encourage caregivers who are comfortable with prayer to make sure they build prayer into their daily routine. Prayer is also a way to connect with your care recipient.

I will never forget the time that I arrived to visit my mother in the nursing home and I could not find her anywhere. Frustrated and a bit unnerved, I asked one of her caregivers where she might be. She said, "Oh your mom is in the chapel." I was shocked. My mother was not particularly religious and never found religion particularly soothing or engaging. When I walked into the synagogue, I saw my mother sitting in the front pew, looking at the beautiful stained glass, and sort of appearing as if she were in deep prayer. I quietly sat next to her and asked her why she was there. She quietly shared, "I was praying to God, asking him to help me understand why I am so forgetful." I turned to her and asked her if she thought he would answer her and she said yes. She mentioned she prayed to him a lot. I then asked her if she would like to pray with me. She said yes, and I held her hand and we prayed together. It is a memory that I will never forget.

For many caregivers, prayer has been a very integral part of their lives. Yet, some of you may not have thought about sharing prayer with your care recipient. I hope the above example will inspire you to consider doing so.

Religion and Spirituality

> Hope is the pillar of the world.
> —Kanuri tribe, *A Tiny Treasure of African Proverbs*

This section is primarily for those of you who see yourselves as religious or spiritual people. If this describes you, most likely you experience great comfort from your religious and spiritual communities. Many of your rituals also provide comfort, yet a number of caregivers who are religious have shared with me that they often don't attend their places of worship because of time. They are so busy caring for their care recipient that they have no time for anything else, even attending their place of worship. Others have shared they didn't participate in religious events because they couldn't take their care recipient with them. Still others lost faith in their religious beliefs. In my experience, I have found just a small number of caregivers who are able to attend their place of worship on a regular basis.

Now is the time you need the support of a community. It can keep you grounded and ease your caregiving journey. By doing so, you can reap many gifts and blessings in return. And if you cannot physically get to your places of worship, you may gain comfort through praying, reading the message of the day, or enjoy reading a bible passage.

In the case of care recipients who have dementia, oftentimes their recollection of prayers, stories, and hymns is very much intact. You may find that singing hymns or other religious or spiritual songs can help you connect. I am truly grateful for the many religious and spiritual beliefs, prayers, songs, and rituals I took advantage of while my mother was ill. I urge you to reconnect with your spirituality or place of worship. Making the time to participate can be important to your overall health and well-being.

Being Mindful of Your Body

Not only can caregiving deplete your spirit and cause emotional distress, it can deplete your energy, weaken your body's immune system, and affect your overall well-being. Often, caregivers operate in high gear and aren't even aware of how much their body is being taxed. Unfortunately, it is not until your care recipient dies or you become sick that you are aware of such stress. The following are some ideas and exercises that you can use to become more mindful about your body. Remember, your body is with you wherever you go and whatever you do. If you listen and pay attention to the signals your body gives, you'll be better able to take care of yourself.

Nourishing your Body

Nourishing your body with balanced meals and proper hydration is important. Too often, you may not eat well because you are exhausted and the idea of fixing a meal is overwhelming. It's not unusual for caregivers to eat on the run or snack their way through each day. Yet it is important to eat foods that nourish and replenish you. Here are suggestions for having healthier foods available to you:

- Plan a half day, your "nourishing food day," where you cook meals for the week. Maybe even ask a few friends to cook with you. Make it fun if you can. Consider cooking large quantities so you can freeze them for dinners and lunches.
- In order to have the time to cook uninterrupted, you may need to ask a friend, family member, neighbor, or church member to take care of your care recipient.
- Consider hiring a food preparation service or purchasing prepared food, which can reduce the burden of cooking for yourself or your family.

And for the physical care of your body:

Your body isn't able to take care of itself without some love and attention. You have to "check in" with your body every so often. Consider these questions:

- How tired is your body? Do you get at least six hours of sleep a night, or do you rest or meditate during the day?
- Is your body well nourished with food and hydration?
- Do you take the time to make sure you drink enough fluids throughout the day?
- Are you eating at least two healthy meals a day to replenish yourself?

Do you listen to what your body tells you?

- Are you having pain, palpitations, soreness, stiffness, sluggishness, or exhaustion?
- Do you get sick often?
- Have you gained or lost weight?
- Do you have constant headaches or backaches?

- Do you ever give your body a gift? This can be whatever makes you feel good, but it must be healthy for you, such as a massage, chiropractic adjustment, whirlpool bath, yoga, tai chi, or water aerobics.

How you answer the above questions can provide a glimpse into what areas of your health you need to attend to. Below are some suggestions for taking care of your body and having fun in the process:

- Engage in an activity that you enjoy (if you can get a friend to join you, that's even better)
- Take a relaxing bath
- Play in the garden
- Take walks outside by yourself or with someone if you prefer company
- Dance
- Participate in yoga or tai chi
- Consider or continue to engage in exercise, such as swimming, biking, or hiking

Once you practice being mindful about your body, I hope you will feel better and will want to continue to take care of it. One last point that deserves your attention: Be sure to get routine physicals and go to the doctor when you aren't feeling well. If you don't take care of yourself physically, you won't be able to take care of your care recipient.

Humor and Laughter

> Like a welcome summer rain, humor may suddenly cleanse and cool the earth, the air and you.
>
> —Langston Hughes, *The Book of Negro Humor*, 7

Some of you may be surprised that I am including a section on humor and laughter. However, for many caregivers, the ability to laugh and keep a sense of humor helped ease their way and balance some of the sad and more difficult times.

The book *Anatomy of an Illness* by Norman Cousins and Rene Dubos points to the healing effects of humor during stressful times.[3] Cousins wrote this book after being diagnosed with ankylosing spondylitis, a serious illness that attacks the connective tissues of the body. At the time, he was the editor of the *Saturday Review* and felt that stress played a great part in his illness. During a hospital stay, he began to research the effects of stress on the body and the immune system. Feeling that the hospital was a stressful place, he checked himself out of the hospital and into a hotel. He hired a nurse, read humorous stories, and they watched Marx Brothers' movies together. Amazingly he recovered. To this day, there are many people who don't believe this story. I believe he was onto something very important. There exists quite a bit of research that has been done on laughter and the positive effects on health.

The following bullet points are from the Mayo Clinic's research on laughter.[4] Similar findings about the importance of laughter and humor have been found in research studies worldwide.

Stress Relief from Laughter

While humor can't cure all ailments, there is increased evidence about the positive aspects of laughter. Laughter can:

- Stimulate your heart, lungs, and muscles, and increase endorphins in your brain
- Clear the tension in your body and help calm you
- Help relax your muscles and reduce some of the physical symptoms of stress

Long-Term Effects of Laughter

Laughter works short term but can also be good for your long-term health and well-being. Laughter can:

- Improve your immune system, help fight stress and potentially more-serious illnesses
- Cause the body to produce its own natural painkillers

Laughter can help you cope with difficult situations. I will always remember the visits with my mother when we would watch the *I Love Lucy* and *Golden Girls* comedy shows. It felt so good to laugh together and helped offset some of the more frustrating and sad times. As a way of taking care of my spirit, I made it a habit to watch something funny every night before going to sleep. I still practice this ritual almost daily.

I remember a very dear, special time with one of my clients whose husband was dying. I went with her to the nursing home to see her husband. She asked to talk with me privately as she had had a particularly rough day. Our conversation started out serious as she was describing her day. As she continued to share, I helped her see some of the funny aspects of her situation. We ended up laughing so hard we both had tears coming from our eyes. Her husband died soon after. She shared that our time together just laughing the day before her husband died was a time she will always remember. She said that she so needed to laugh to relieve some of her sadness and grief.

I hope that after reading this section some of you can find a way to bring humor and laughter into your journey. Humor and laughter can "cleanse the soul."

Creating a Circle of Support

The caregiving journey can be a long road. People tend to be there for you in the beginning, but then as time goes on, they begin to drift away. The long-term aspects of chronic illness can be isolating.

One of the most helpful ways I took care of myself during my mother's Alzheimer's disease was creating what I call a "circle of support." A circle of support is composed of people and activities that support you and fill your emotional well. In other words, your circle should be a soothing and calming influence. Your circle of support needs to be chosen carefully and thoughtfully. I chose people and activities that filled my spirit in positive ways. I also became more aware of the people and activities that depleted my spirit—and quite frankly, I began to let go of those people and activities. My circle of support was made up of family, friends, colleagues, and activities that supported me, made me laugh, and were low maintenance. My activities and hobbies were ones that made me feel good and didn't add stress. I was very mindful of making sure I had a "circle of support" throughout my caregiving journey. My circle of support was absolutely essential to my overall health and well-being throughout my journey with my mother.

In my practice, I have emphasized to caregivers the importance of creating a circle of support. Caring for someone with Alzheimer's disease or other chronic illnesses can easily deplete you. It's important to find ways to nurture you. In many caregiving situations, your care recipient is unable to be in a reciprocal relationship because of his or her illness. As the caregiver, you give much of yourself and do not get much back. Caregivers have shared with me how helpful it was for them to have a circle of support. When working with caregivers, I suggest they diagram their circle of support on paper. They are amazed at how many of their circles are filled with people or activities that drained their spirits or that they don't have circles to fill.

Identifying the supports that exist and the areas of support that need to be developed can encourage you to take better care of yourself. The most important aspect of creating a circle of support is making sure that your circles are available and provide support, nurturance, and relief.

Before I share some case examples illustrating how circles of support can be helpful, let's look at how to diagram on paper what your circle of support might look like. To begin, draw a circle in the middle of your paper. Place your name in that circle. That circle represents you. Then draw a number of circles around your circle. Those circles represent your various sources of support, which can be people, activities, or other things that bring you comfort. For example, you may draw a circle that represents your family. Another circle might represent your favorite activity, and so forth.

Below are some case examples of how caregivers have utilized the circle of support. One is of an adult daughter, and the other, a spouse. What is critical in this exercise is not only identifying your circles of support, but then being aware of which circles support you and which deplete you. In addition, if you have mostly empty circles, it is now time to begin to fill them in with supports that can be helpful to you.

Karen's Circle of Support

Karen: An Adult Daughter

Karen was referred to me because she was feeling overwhelmed. She came to the first session sharing that she felt that she was at a breaking point. Karen was an only child, married with two teenagers, and worked part time. Her father had died ten years earlier. Her mom insisted on staying in her own home after her husband died. While Karen wasn't thrilled with that choice, she respected her mother's right to make her own decisions. Her mother had been doing pretty well until about a year earlier, when she fell and broke her hip. However, after her mother finished her physical therapy, she wanted to go back to her home. Karen wasn't pleased but continued to support her mother's decision. Yet the past year had been quite challenging for Karen. Karen was continually receiving phone calls from her mother, needing her help. Her mother denied this. I explained to Karen that she was serving as her mother's

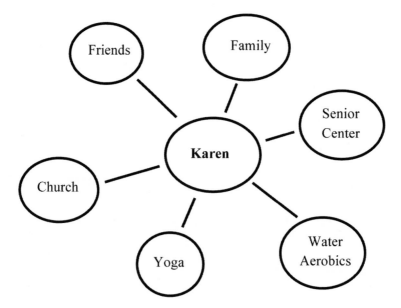

Figure 4.1. Karen's Circle of Support

"care manager." She was, in effect, managing all her care, which caused her to feel overwhelmed and drained. Karen's own spirit was being depleted since she was the lone person responsible for taking care of her mother.

We discussed the importance of creating a circle of support so that she wasn't the sole caregiver. Karen needed relief, and Karen's mother needed others in her life besides her daughter. The first circle involved reaching out to her mother's church. We were able to find people who could bring meals, visit with her mother, and take her to appointments. The second circle involved connecting her mother to a senior center where she could get valuable social interaction from other seniors. The third circle for her mother involved expanding the network of family members and friends who could help when needed in order to relieve Karen of some of the responsibility.

At first, Karen was hesitant. She didn't think her extended family would help as they were quite busy themselves. She also didn't want to bother her friends. I was able to help her let go of the belief that only she could be available. I encouraged Karen to think about various tasks that could be assigned to others. Within a month, Karen began to feel balanced and less overwhelmed. She was quite amazed at how willing and supportive her friends and family were.

Next, we created some new circles of support for Karen, personally. We looked at her friends. Karen quickly recognized which friends were able to really be there for her. She was particularly interested in surrounding herself with people who made her laugh and gave her happiness. Next, we created a circle of support that would foster more ease and help relieve some of her stress. She decided it would be important for her to go back to her yoga and water aerobics classes. Lastly, I encouraged her to be involved in doing fun things with her family. She began watching popular sitcoms with her teenage kids, went to comedy shows and movies with her husband, and tried to find activities that would bring her joy and fun.

Dan: A Spousal Caregiver

Dan was eighty years old and married. His wife had early onset dementia but was quite capable of taking care of herself. Yet, because of her forgetfulness, Dan was uncomfortable with her cooking for them. They had one daughter, Sara, who was fifty years old and had been disabled much of her life. She lived with Dan and his wife. Dan, however, began to realize he was becoming overwhelmed trying to attend to his wife and oversee Sara's increasing medical needs. In fact, Dan took Sara to the emergency room at least once a month. Additionally, Dan had been diagnosed with a pretty serious heart condition. Given his wife's dementia, she was unable to help or care for Dan or Sara.

Dan was referred to me by his elder law attorney. His elder law attorney was concerned that Dan was emotionally and physically worn out. He felt Dan needed to have a plan in place in case something were to happen to him. After many tension-filled meetings with Dan, his wife, and Sara, we developed an action plan to find a suitable living environment that could provide Sara the type of care she required. Fortunately, they were in a good financial position, which enabled Dan to secure a small, one-room apartment.

Now that Dan had found a safe place for Sara to live, I explained to Dan that he needed some relief from being the sole caregiver to her. We developed a circle of support to provide for Sara. This would be particularly important if he were to die. A meeting was set up with the retirement community director to discuss what the next steps would be as Sara continued to decline. We developed a plan of care together that would support Sara down the road.

The next circle of support was to connect Dan and Sara to a small home care agency that could be available in an emergency. This agency could send a caregiver to accompany Sara to the hospital and serve as her advocate. After much encouragement, Dan began to let go of being the sole caregiver. The last circle involved finding a church that was willing to provide friendly visitors to Sara. They not only provided Sara some companionship but also served as additional eyes and ears and were able to report any concerns they saw when they visited. If Dan hadn't had the financial resources to move Sara to a care community, I would have helped him create circles of support that would have provided him some relief at home.

After I helped Dan set up a circle of support around his daughter, I strongly encouraged Dan to create a circle of support for himself. We connected with his church and they agreed to help. I also helped Dan find someone who could act as power of attorney if he became ill or died. We discussed what types of supports he might need if he became frail or incapacitated. This was the hardest for Dan, because he was not used to considering himself.

While Dan had resources, not everyone does. When families have limited finances, I look at creative options and engage community resources as much as possible, such as churches, synagogues, neighbors, college students, and aging services resources.

My hope is that this chapter has provided you with many different ways to support yourself so that you can take better care of you. In chapter 6, "Navigating the Maze of Resources, Services, and Support," I provide several other ways to take care of yourself so you feel less isolated. Remember, the most important aspect of self-care is committing to the belief that you matter too.

NOTES

1. Faith S. Luyster, Patrick J. Strollo, Phyllis C. Zee, and James K. Walsh, "Sleep: A Health Imperative," *Sleep* 35, no. 6 (2012).

2. Jack Kornfield, *A Path with a Heart: A Guide through the Perils and Promises of Spiritual Life* (New York: Bantam Books, 1993), 20.

3. Norman Cousins and Rene Dubos, *Anatomy of an Illness as Perceived by the Patient: Reflections on Healing and Regeneration* (New York: W. W. Norton, 1979).

4. Mayo Clinic, "Stress Relief from Laughter? Yes, No Joke," www.mayoclinic.com/health/stress-relief/SR00034/.

FIVE

Inspiring More Meaningful Engagement

Finding Ways to Be Together

All things are possible to him who believes.

—Mark 9:23

I was inspired to write this chapter because of the hundreds of caregivers who have asked how to best communicate with their elder family members or care recipients who have lost the ability to communicate verbally. Caregivers find this situation particularly difficult and are challenged to find different ways to engage and relate. Many chronic diseases cause continual loss of verbal abilities, and various forms of dementia make it difficult to connect because the care recipient no longer has access to his memories. Thus caregivers have to find new ways to accommodate and adjust to the unending changes. As a mindful caregiver, your goal is to communicate with intention and compassion. This chapter explains the barriers to communication and provides new ways to connect with your care recipient. It is hoped that this information will put you more at ease.

UNDERSTANDING COMMUNICATION

Communication has always been at the heart and center of relationships and one of the major ways we engage with one another. It is one of the complicated aspects of human behavior and can keep people engaged or cut off from one another. Communication is one of the most important skills we learn because it:

- Keeps us connected to one another

- Helps get our needs met
- Helps us remain more independent
- Allows us to express thoughts and feelings

There are many factors that can affect the communication between you and your care recipient:

- The environment where the communication is taking place. For example, is the environment too loud or is there too much stimuli? These can be distracting and overwhelming to your care recipient.
- The content of the information and whether it is appropriate for the person with whom you are communicating.
- Whether you are communicating clearly.
- How the communication is expressed, such as your tone of voice, facial expressions, and body language.
- Whether you are more interested in making a point or being right than you are about being understood.
- The timing of the communication; for example, is the care recipient too tired to be able to listen to what you are saying?
- Whether the person is willing to listen and receive what you are trying to share.
- How the information is perceived or interpreted. People have their own lens through which they perceive and interpret information.
- How much the person is able to understand cognitively and emotionally.

Interestingly, while communicating verbally is most often the preferred method, up to 80 percent of the way we communicate is nonverbal. We learn nonverbal communication right out of the womb. As infants, when we were hungry, thirsty, or tired, we communicated in a variety of ways, such as by fidgeting, grimacing, or making faces. Our caregivers had to figure out what we were trying to say or what we needed. And most adults, particularly parents, became experts at figuring out our nonverbal behaviors. Yet most adults communicate verbally, so when another adult cannot communicate with her words, we can find it frustrating, confusing, and challenging. Somehow the patience we managed when trying to understand infants and young children may be missing with adults who can't express themselves verbally.

Aside from the communication challenges, caregivers also struggle with how to maintain a positive relationship with their care recipient. Finding meaningful ways to engage can help caregivers feel more connected to the experience of caregiving. The following section will hopefully provide you with some new insights and increased understanding of how to best communicate with your care recipient.

ENGAGEMENT—THE GREAT DIVIDE

> The trouble is, old age is not interesting until one gets there. It's a foreign country with an unknown language to the young and even middle-aged.
>
> —May Sarton, *As We Are Now*, 23

There appears to be a "great divide" when caregivers from the younger generation attempt to communicate and engage with care recipients of the older generation. Those individuals born from 1926 to 1944 are known as the "Silent" or "Traditionalist" generation. The Traditionalists lived as youth through the Great Depression and the lingering political changes in work and the economic and social policies that followed. These experiences helped shape their attitudes about family, life, and work. As a group, they tend to value hard work, sacrifice, dedication, frugality, and duty before pleasure. The experiences of the Traditionalist generation can pose a number of obstacles that can get in the way of their getting the care and services they need. This can wreak havoc between the caregiver and care recipient. For example, those from the older generation tend to be much more private and less comfortable sharing their emotions and feelings. They may become unwilling to go to a counselor or attend a support group. In addition, they often are not willing to share financial, medical, or other personal information with their family caregivers because they believe it is "their personal business" and often won't allow their children to become involved.

In her book *Another Country*, Mary Pipher discusses how vastly different the social, emotional, physical, financial, and environmental landscapes are for the Traditionalist care recipients.[1] The word *landscape* is used deliberately to highlight elders' "different perspectives and life experiences." She points out that this generation feels as if they came from "another country."[2] In my experience as a therapist, I would have to agree. There is no doubt that the behavior and choices elders make during their lives have been greatly influenced by these perspectives. I bring this to the reader's attention, because understanding this generation can provide insight into how to best engage with them regarding care. In my practice, I have found that difficult relationships between adult children caregivers and elders often result from these generational differences.

As caregivers to this older generation, it will take some compassion and patience to conquer this great divide. I share the following case example to help caregivers better understand these generational challenges. These challenges are not easy, even for therapists, as I had to learn to overcome them as well. And I will admit that, at times, they have felt like insurmountable differences.

The Emotional Terrain

The best way to describe how the emotional terrain can be so different for the older generation is with the following example:

The Great Depression: Karen and Belle

Karen had brought her eighty-five-year-old mother, Belle, to my office because she was concerned about her mother's depression. When Karen would try to talk with Belle about her depression, her mother would become angry and say she had no idea what depression was! I began my session with both of them by asking Belle if she could share how she felt. It was clear that she had a hard time expressing her feelings. Her answers to my questions, as well as her behavior and affect, indicated she was indeed depressed. Yet when I tried to give this feedback to Belle, she quickly retorted, "Karen thinks I'm depressed, but I am not crazy." In the same breath, she went on, "In fact, the only depression I have faced was the Great Depression." Belle went on to say, "Karen has no idea how bad it was living back then; nothing can compare."

It was clear that Belle saw herself as a survivor. Often, this generation used the word *depression* in the context of the Great Depression, and that they also equate being depressed with being crazy. Over the years, I have encountered numerous examples of how different the members of the Traditionalist generation experienced their emotional terrain. They believe that life is supposed to be difficult and you must learn to live with whatever comes your way. Their expectations about how to live life are quite different from the younger generation. Their mantra seems to be, "Life is not a bed of roses." They keep their emotions and feelings to themselves. Also, remember that during their lifetime, counseling, for the longest time, was not even available; when it did become more acceptable and commonplace, they were very reluctant to use it.

Many elders have echoed Belle's sentiment: If they have to go to a counselor, it means they are crazy. So instead of asking elders if they are depressed, I ask if they feel sad, lonely, or angry. This language shift has been rather effective in helping elders sort out their feelings. They have been much more receptive to interventions to help them cope with their depression. I share this example because, as caregivers, you too need to recognize that the emotional terrain has to be traversed very sensitively and carefully.

The Physical Terrain

The physical terrain is another area that can greatly impact how caregivers communicate with their care recipients. The physical terrain describes the various environments in which elders grew up and includes their neighborhoods, workplaces, and religious communities. Many elders grew up in towns in which everybody knew everybody, and everyone supported each other. Oftentimes, their religious institutions were a vital part of their existence, and from which they drew much comfort and companionship. And unlike subsequent generations, Traditionalists grew up among multigenerational families. In many cases, it was not unusual to have cousins, aunts, uncles, and grandparents in the same household or at least in the same community.

However, as society changed, people moved for jobs, and technological advances changed the old way of life, the physical terrain changed as well. Many people began taking jobs far away and neighborhoods began to change. Thus, their social lives and networks of support became less available.

I believe the physical terrain of the twenty-first century has made it much more difficult for caregivers and care recipients. For one, many adult children live away from their elder family members, and figuring out how best to provide help and support is challenging. "Caring at a distance," as this is called by gerontologists, can cause worry, concern, and a great deal of stress for caregivers. Secondly, managing the logistics from a distance creates additional stress. Caregivers often have to take time off work and leave their own families in order to help. Thirdly, caregivers ultimately struggle with the decision to physically move the elder closer to themselves or another family member. And the elders often have a hard time recognizing how these changes have impacted their functioning and way of relating to others. Time and again, when the elder and adult children begin the conversations about the best living arrangements for the elder, I hear the same lament, "I don't need to move and if I need help my neighbors will help me." Elders tend to hold onto their memories of how life used to be or have some denial about their situation. Thus the physical environment can present numerous challenges that require careful and thoughtful planning.

"I Can't Sleep at Night" — A Long-Distance Daughter and Her Father

Carole called me because she said she didn't know what to do about her father's situation. He was eighty-five years old and had been living alone in the home he and his wife shared for over forty years. His wife had died two years earlier. She was the social connector of the family and also made sure his needs were met. Since her death, her father had basically isolated himself. He stayed in his home all day and went out only once a day for his lunch meal. He had lost weight because he didn't eat properly and seemed uninterested in life. In addition, he had a serious heart condition. However, what tipped Carole over the edge was when she learned her father had fallen and hit his head but refused to go to the ER. "That was the last straw," Carole said to me. "I can't stand it anymore. I wake up at night worrying about him. I try to visit as much as possible, at least four to five times a year. But it's not enough. How do I convince him he needs to move closer to me and his grandchildren?"

Unfortunately, situations like this are more common than not. Long-distance caregiving can be difficult and nerve-wracking to say the least. Certainly from Carole's father's perspective, it's understandable that he would rather remain in his own home. And up to then, no matter what Carole said to him, he said he just wanted to stay in his own home.

In situations such as this, when you have an older adult who is competent but not making the safest choices for himself, you can't really force him to move. However, the following were ideas I presented to Carole:

- Carole could *go with his resistance* and instead of pushing him to move, validate how fortunate he has been to still live in his home. Carole could have a conversation with him and tell him that she understands he doesn't want to leave his home and community; however, might he be willing to visit her and the grandchildren more frequently and for longer visits? This suggestion helps validate his feelings and tugs at his heartstrings, as he loves his grandchildren.
- Carole might consider *contacting the doctor* her father has the best relationship with and see if that doctor would be willing to recommend assisted living care. If he respects the doctor and the doctor takes a strong position about his moving, this could potentially move him at least into a safer place.
- Carole might think about a *role her father could be a part of* in their family life, if he moved to Atlanta. For example, if her father could feel as if he were needed he might be more inclined to move. Carole's father had a woodworking hobby and perhaps he could teach his grandson (who was in college) woodworking. The grandson agreed and began to talk to his grandfather about their spending some summer time together.

Fortunately, when his grandson invited him to visit over the summer, he accepted. In addition, Carole was able to get him to build bird houses that he could present as gifts to various nursing homes in the area. Within six months, Carole and her family were able to talk him into moving, and he agreed.

However, for every situation that is successful there can be another that is not. When the older adult is competent and refuses to move, you, as the adult child, have to step back and hope for the best.

The Financial Terrain

Lastly, this section would not be complete without discussing the financial terrain, which is how elders approach money. This issue tends to be one of the most exasperating for adult caregivers, as critical decisions cannot be made without a thorough understanding of the elder's financial situation. Remember that many elders came over from other countries with little or nothing and were also influenced by the Depression. Traditionalists tend to save money and spend it cautiously. They also lived for quite some time without credit cards. For many, the idea of not paying for something right away is a foreign concept. Because many elders lost a lot of money during the Depression, trust has always played a significant role in how elders have dealt with their money. I have heard many stories of elders who would hide their money in their mattresses or keep it in hidden places in their homes. They only spent what they had. So trying to have the financial planning conversations can be fraught with stress, tension, and frustration. To help caregivers cope with this aspect of caregiving, the following is a very common example and presents some ideas on how to navigate this difficult terrain.

"I Am Not Stupid"—Mildred and Her Daughter Sarah

Sarah called for a consult because she was very worried about her mother. Sarah had begun to notice that her mother's short-term memory was failing. Mildred would repeat herself often and seemed to become easily confused and overwhelmed. Mildred's finances were fairly limited. Mildred was still in charge of all her finances except for her brokerage account. Part of Sarah's weekly visit with her mother was to check her mail and bills. In doing so, she began noticing that Mildred was receiving a great many solicitations from churches and other organizations. She wondered how many of these organizations Mildred gave contributions to. One day on her visit with Mildred, she decided to ask her mother about them. Mildred became very defensive and said, "Do you think I am stupid? I know who I give to!" Sarah was not so convinced. She was quite concerned that her mother was not aware to whom and how much she was giving away. Sarah found an opportunity to look through her checkbook and noticed several thousand dollars' worth of checks that had been written over the past six months. Knowing that Mildred had limited funds, Sarah became quite worried. She felt she might need to take over Mildred's checkbook and finances. Yet she was at a loss as to how to approach her mother.

I present this case example, as it is a rather common one. As a mindful caregiver, a thoughtful approach must be sensitive to all the generational issues at play. For elders, financial issues can also affect the emotional and physical terrains. As a result, the combination can often create a wedge between the adult children and the elder. Addressing these concerns requires caregivers to tackle this in small steps whenever possible. In Sarah's situation, I encouraged her to address the *least threatening issue* first and then go after the more difficult issues later.

Sarah and I felt that the least threatening issue for her to tackle would be the organization of solicitations. Sarah's challenge was to try to limit the number of organizations that were soliciting Mildred and to determine together how many Mildred would give to. I suggested the following:

- First, Sarah needed to find a way to help her mother feel as much in control as possible. Plus, it was important that Mildred feel she was still contributing to society. Many care recipients feel that their adult children treat them like children. They want to feel like they not only still have some control in their lives but that they are also contributing members of their society.
- Next, instead of telling her mother she was donating too much money (which Mildred had denied and most likely would still deny), I suggested she talk with her mother about choosing three or four organizations each year that she could donate to. Then Sarah would encourage Mildred to decide how much she would like to give.
- Third, I suggested they come up with a schedule of when Mildred would write the checks and place the dates on a calendar. It was important that Mildred still write the checks herself.
- I also suggested that Sarah get her mother's permission to collect and file the other solicitation mail. That way, Mildred could look in the file at a later point in time and choose organizations to which she could donate. Again, the purpose of this was to help Mildred still feel like she was in control.

The next issue was much more challenging, talking with Mildred about becoming her POA for finances. Sarah did not yet have Mildred's power of attorney (POA) for finances. This is a difficult issue, as many elders don't fully understand what is meant by a POA for finances and falsely believe that they lose their rights and control. Additionally, when a care recipient has short-term memory problems, they can become paranoid, which makes matters worse. In Sarah's situation, because her mother had memory issues, it was critical that Sarah talk with Mildred right away before her memory became even worse. Mildred was still able to understand what a POA meant, even though her generational issues and personality made it challenging for her to accept. After several conversations, Mildred agreed to give Sarah her POA.

Establishing a POA for an elder can be a sensitive issue and often goes against the very grain of how elders feel about privacy and independence. Many elders will dig their heels in the sand and refuse to talk about this topic. Others may discuss it but still refuse to do anything. The following are a few ideas provided for Sarah that may also be helpful to you.

Idea One

Think about who might be the *best person* to begin the discussion of what a POA is and how that he or she could be helpful to your care recipient. Sometimes that person may be a clergy member, accountant or lawyer, grandchild or good friend. It is critical in this first conversation for the care recipient not to feel threatened. So often care recipients think the caregiver is trying to take over and gain control. One way to approach this is to ask who your care recipient would want to be in charge if there were an emergency and she needed someone to take over for her. The operative word is *emergency*, as this word often feels less threatening and gives the impression that the POA would only be needed in the future.

Idea Two

Another suggestion is to state that you are getting a POA and ask your care recipient if she has one as well. In Sarah's instance, she could ask Mildred if she would consider getting a POA together. I have found this idea works quite well. Interestingly, many caregivers don't have POAs either and they need to!

Idea Three

If your care recipient absolutely refuses to discuss why a POA is important and how it could help her, then you may need to enlist the help of the care recipient's physician. I have found that some doctors are willing to have this conversation in the office with their patient to include the health care POA along with the financial POA. Of course, not every physician will be willing to do this.

Idea Four

When all else fails, you may have to revert to presenting a therapeutic lie. A therapeutic lie should only be used with the help of a professional and when the elder is in an unsafe situation. Essentially, a therapeutic lie is a sort of white lie. (See chapter 2 for a more thorough discussion of this issue.) In Sarah's situation, the therapeutic lie would entail telling Mildred that, if she were to have a sudden stroke and couldn't take care of her personal affairs, without a POA, the government could take over and make financial decisions for her. I have found that many elders of Mildred's generation don't want the government to get their money.

In Sarah's situation, she convinced her mother to let her keep a second eye on her finances, but winning her mother's approval to sign the POA was another story. After several months of help from Mildred's doctor and minister, she finally conceded. There can be situations in which the elder may not concede. If the elder is in a dangerous situation, such as vulnerable to being taken advantage of, the only next step would be to consider guardianship.

COMMUNICATION AND CONNECTION IN THE TWENTY-FIRST CENTURY

The Internet and New Media

The twenty-first century has introduced new ways in which people communicate and engage with one another. The Internet and social media has connected and some would say disconnected people of all generations. For many elders, this new way of communicating feels foreign and uncomfortable. For others, the Internet has been life transforming and a great way to stay connected to family, friends, and events of the world. However, a good many people seventy-five-plus are not comfortable with the Internet, and for those who are, many are not particularly media savvy. They find these new forms of communication both challenging and imposing. Many elders have shared with me that they are not happy with the ways their relationships with the younger members in their families, including their adult children, have changed.

There seems to be one main complaint—elders feel their family members are so involved in their smartphones, devices, and computers that they don't get their full time and attention. The following case example is of an elder who felt like a "second fiddle" to her daughter's smartphone.

"Second Fiddle"—Martha and Her Daughter Jane

Martha and her daughter Jane came to me because they were continually frustrated with what they called their "lack of communication and understanding" of one another. Martha was particularly upset, as she mentioned that she and Jane had always had a close relationship. Martha shared that she looked forward to spending time with her daughter. However, things changed when her daughter bought her smartphone. Martha said she now feels "second fiddle" to her daughter's devices. Martha explained that on many occasions when they were together, during the middle of her conversation with Jane, Jane would be interrupted by a text message or e-mail. She said Jane would immediately turn her attention to her phone and forget she was present. She went on to further say that it seemed as if Jane were more interested in spending time on her devices than with her. Martha also felt that her daughter was not aware of how upsetting this was to her. When I turned to Jane for her perspective, she became somewhat defensive, saying she does not always answer her text messages or e-mails when they are together. She felt like her mother was blowing this way out of proportion. Plus, she mentioned she was tired of hearing her mother complain about how computers and devices were ruining everyone's lives.

After they expressed their feelings, they recognized what was most upsetting was that they were not happy about how they were relating to one another. They also realized each was blaming the other and harboring anger. Martha and Jane realized they wanted to be mindful of being "fully present" with one another. They decided that when they were together, unless it was an emergency situation, Jane would not answer her phone or use her devices when she was with her mother. Her mother agreed to not complain about how the Internet is ruining her children's and grandchildren's lives. They took the time to really listen to each other and pushed their judgments aside. This helped them to both feel more at ease again in their relationship.

On the positive side, many elders use e-mail to keep in touch with their family, friends, and even doctors. Some elders are even more tech savvy and stay connected to adult children and grandchildren by using Skype or Facetime, which are programs that allow a person to communicate via a camera connected to a computer. The following is an example of a positive influence of the Internet.

"Fly the Friendly Internet Skies of Skype" —
Sylvia and Her Granddaughter Ellen

Sylvia's physician referred her to me because she was not eating much, didn't want to socialize with her friends, and was depressed. Unfortunately, her antidepressant medication didn't seem to be helping. Less than a year earlier, Sylvia had lost her only daughter, and her granddaughter Ellen was about to be married. Sylvia was sad that her daughter would not be present at Ellen's wedding. However, her main issue was that she was extremely upset about not being able to attend her granddaughter's wedding either. She told me she could not make the long plane ride to Seattle from Atlanta as her arthritis rendered it difficult for her to be very mobile. She mentioned she and Ellen were quite close and even more so since her daughter's death. I asked Sylvia how she stayed in touch with Ellen and she said mostly by telephone and sometimes e-mail.

It then occurred to me that there might be several ways to help Sylvia feel more a part of the wedding. I suggested that she and Ellen set up a video connection using Skype or other such program. That way, Ellen could "model" her dress for Sylvia and Sylvia would be able to see her live. I encouraged Ellen to think of other ways Sylvia could feel part of the wedding. Ellen rose to the occasion and found many creative ways to share her wedding preparations. Sylvia was tickled to no end. Ellen also videotaped her wedding so that Sylvia could see the whole ceremony. Sylvia was elated and felt so grateful her whole demeanor changed.

There is no doubt that the Internet has greatly changed the ways people communicate with one another. These changes can further the disconnection between the young and old or be used in positive ways to bring additional joy and connection.

OUR INDEPENDENT DRIVEN CULTURE

The irony of life is that we enter and leave this world dependent on those who love us.

Our culture's strong emphasis on independence is another issue that impacts connection. Historically, we have been a communal people, recognizing that our very survival depended on one another. Being a "we" or "they" was valued and expected. However, particularly as society has evolved in this century, "we" and "they" have been substituted by "I." Most of us strive to be "independent." Many care recipients will go to great lengths to not be a burden, even if it places them in precariously unsafe situations. The idea of being a burden is to be avoided at all costs. And that ethic is reinforced in every aspect of our lives. Ram Dass in his book *Still Here* provides an interesting perspective on this fierce sense of independence.[3] He believes people would be better served if they could learn to become what he calls "joyfully dependent." Being joyfully dependent requires being willing to ask for help or support in order to remain as independent as possible. I call this interdependence, which is the intersection of dependency and independency. It paves the way for learning to be joyfully dependent. It's important for caregivers to discuss interdependence, as it allows new opportunities for engagement for both caregivers and care recipients.

"I Am Fine, Thank You" — Gertrude and Son, Marcus

Marcus called me in desperation about getting help for his mother, Gertrude, who was in her late eighties. Marcus noticed several troubling changes, including that his mother was becoming increasingly forgetful, was not keeping up with medications, and was not eating well on her own. When Marcus suggested getting a caregiver for her, Gertrude quickly responded, "I am fine, thank you. I do not need any help." When I met with them both, Marcus again stated that he felt that Gertrude needed assistance. Gertrude quickly retorted that she comes from strong German stock and knows how to take care of herself. She denied that she needed any help with meal preparation or medication management. She proudly shared how she was a writer and had to be meticulously organized and that she still was. When Marcus confronted Gertrude with her short-term memory issues, she said, "All older people have some memory issues."

Given Gertrude's pride and independence, I knew Marcus would not be able to convince her that she needed help. In circumstances in which an elder care recipient is either in denial or isn't truly aware of her situation, it's best to not argue. This tact often gets you nowhere. Instead, I suggested that Marcus reinforce Gertrude's independence, with the idea being that Marcus needed to first build a bridge of validation and respect. The next step would be to introduce a caregiver into the mix. Matching Gertrude to someone who could seem more like a companion would be essential. Fortunately, I was able to find a German caregiver who was introduced as a friend whom Marcus had met at his church. At first, the caregiver would take Gertrude out to lunch. It turned out that Gertrude ended up enjoying the company of this caregiver. As Gertrude became more at ease, the caregiver began cooking her meals and helping her with her medications. This situation turned out in a positive way, but unfortunately, not all do. The rule of thumb should be that if the care recipient is in danger of harming herself or others, an intervention will need to take place without the consent of the care recipient.

HOW CHRONIC DISEASE CAN CREATE DIS-EASE

One goal of the mindful caregiver is to find ways to not feel "diseased" in the caregiving process.

The twenty-first century has introduced some unique issues surrounding communication. More people than in any other century are living into their eighties, nineties, and beyond. Unfortunately, a good many of them are living for years with chronic diseases. Diseases such as cancer, Alzheimer's, and Parkinson's can last for many years and can impact both the caregiver and care recipient. Some of the chronic diseases as those mentioned above can create communication challenges. In most situations, the care recipient's health declines over time. Care recipients may have less energy to sustain engagement. They may also develop more cognitive impairment. Others may be in discomfort, which can make communication difficult. Many care recipients experience a loss of identity and connection with others. They are much more vulnerable to losing their spirit and can easily become withdrawn and depressed.

For caregivers, the challenge is to figure out how to adapt to the health decline of their care recipient so they don't become "dis-eased." I separate the word *disease* into *dis-ease*, to make the point that caring for someone who has a chronic disease can create "dis-ease" if caregivers don't take care of themselves. They can easily become exhausted, and it is not unusual for caregivers to become ill while providing care or soon thereafter. Caregivers' identities also change, as they have to shift their role from an adult child or spouse to caregiver. They have not had to undertake this role previously, so developing new ways to communicate and relate to the care recipient can feel like a daunting task. Yet there are ways to remain engaged and connected and to feel less "dis-eased." The following example will shed light on how caregivers can learn new ways to cope so as to not become "dis-eased."

"Never without Words" — A Wife's Perspective

Joyce came to me because she dreaded having to visit her husband, Jack, at the nursing home. She just didn't know how to communicate with him anymore. He had had a massive stroke and was no longer able to speak, which "was so ironic" as he had been an English professor. Jack, she related, was the author of many books, well read, and a man who loved words. She told me how it just broke her heart to experience him struggling to communicate and how she would often talk for him. Joyce also mentioned how impatient she became with Jack when he tried to communicate something to her. She would end up snapping at him and then feel guilty. It was no wonder that Joyce dreaded her visits.

First, it appeared to me that Joyce had lost the man she knew and had married—the husband who had been so articulate, engaging, and interesting. Essentially, she was grieving over the loss of their shared communication. There is no doubt that Joyce's situation was sad and upsetting for her. Joyce was trying desperately to hold onto the way she remembered her husband and was having a very difficult time letting go of the "old Jack." As long as she held onto this expectation and desire, she would continue to foster anger, resentment, and sadness. She kept hoping that somehow Jack would change and they would be able to communicate the way they used to. Holding this expectation created a negative tension between them.

In order for Joyce to move toward a more comfortable place, she had to acknowledge all her feelings of sadness, anger, and frustration. Then she had to be willing to let go of the old Jack and learn new ways to communicate with him. The following are some ideas I provided to Joyce so she could potentially feel less *dis-eased*.

- Joyce needed to give herself *the space* to grieve and acknowledge her feelings. She had to find a way to quiet her mind to allow her heart to take over. I suggested she build in ten to fifteen minutes each day to meditate or pray. She felt that was doable. As she was able to connect to her heart, she was able to get in touch with her feelings. Once her feelings surfaced, I suggested she just allow herself to "be" with them, acknowledge them, and leave judgment out.
- She also needed to learn to refocus her negative energy and make a conscious effort to energize more positive expressions of her situation. For example, Joyce could write a short story or poem expressing how she felt about the joy her husband's words had given her.

She might be able to recall little sayings or comments that had made her smile.

- Or maybe Joyce could find a way to celebrate her husband's past accomplishments. She could make a donation in his honor, perhaps on his birthday, to the Writers Guild or other literary organization.
- When Joyce visited with him, she could read to him, carefully selecting his favorite book or piece of literature.

Joyce realized that she had never thought of any of these ideas before. She had been so fixated on her anger that she hadn't been willing to let it go. As Joyce began to put some of these suggestions into action, she found her visits were much more pleasant. There were certainly times when she would feel sad. However, she recognized those feelings as normal, allowed herself to feel them, and then let them go so she could be more present with Jack as he was.

"Man's Best Friend"—Joe and His Dog Friends

Joe had a stroke and had recently been placed in a nursing home. He had lost most of his ability to speak in complete sentences, and Joe's children were struggling with how to communicate with him. In the session, Joe's children said that they had agreed to take turns either visiting or calling him every day. When they visited with him, they often found him sitting in his wheelchair with a blank look on his face. He would occasionally acknowledge them by saying hello or just say their name, nothing more. When they visited, they would share what was going on in their lives, but Joe showed little interest. When they tried to talk with him on the phone, he barely uttered a word. They felt frustrated and ready to give up. When I asked his children about Joe's past hobbies, they stated he had few. Then in almost perfect unison, they all said he was a big dog lover. One son had adopted Joe's dog, as the dog wasn't allowed to live in the nursing home. I asked his children if they ever brought Joe's dog to visit. They said no, as they were concerned that a visit from his dog would upset Joe and he would insist that his dog remain with him.

After listening to them, I had several thoughts and ideas for consideration. First, the move was probably confusing and upsetting for Joe. Plus, at some level Joe most likely missed his dog. Perhaps a way to engage Joe might be to introduce dogs into his life. If the visits with other dogs went well, maybe they could eventually bring his dog over for visits. I suggested the following:

- The nursing home had a Happy Tails program, in which therapy dogs were brought into the nursing home to visit with the residents. I suggested they make sure Joe was a part of that program. And I encouraged them to try to visit with him during that activity, if at all possible.

- I often brought along my own dog with me when I was visiting elders, so I asked if I could bring my dog to visit Joe. His family thought that was also a wonderful idea, so my dog also visited Joe.
- In preparing for these dog visits, I recommended they bring a treat box, so that Joe could give dogs treats. Two of his grandchildren decided to make Joe a dog treat box.

Two interesting things happened. After seeing how much joy and comfort Joe received from the dog visits, his children made a great effort to visit him when the Happy Tails program was scheduled. Their visits held more meaning and helped them feel more at ease. Secondly, when they called Joe and asked about dogs, he would actually speak to them in short sentences. They were excited that they had found a topic that seemed to stimulate some conversation.

Now it was time to try to introduce his dog into the visits. The following were some suggestions.

- I had them bring some pictures of his dog and see how he reacted. He enjoyed looking at the pictures but failed to recognize his dog.
- Since he didn't have a negative reaction, I suggested they bring his dog over for a visit and perhaps do so with one of Joe's grandchildren. When his grandson walked in with his grandfather's dog, Joe responded with a big wide grin on his face. He was very happy to see his grandson and the dog.
- Since he didn't remember *his* dog, there wasn't a problem when his grandson left. Ah, the blessing of dementia—sometimes forgetfulness can ease the pain of the loss. From then on, each of his children made every attempt to bring Joe's dog on their visits.

THE UNIQUE COMMUNICATION CHALLENGES WHEN CARE RECIPIENTS HAVE ALZHEIMER'S DISEASE

I felt like I was an archaeologist of the mind, digging for meaning. I dusted off phrases hoping to discover treasures hidden beneath the surfaces of garbled speech.
—Olivia Hoblitzelle, *Ten Thousand Joys & Ten Thousand Sorrows*

Before concluding a discussion on chronic disease and communication, I feel Alzheimer's disease deserves its own separate section. Alzheimer's disease, or AD, has become one of the top ten causes of death in our country.[4] Unfortunately, usual ways of communicating don't necessarily work well with those with AD.

Finding different ways to communicate with care recipients who have AD often eludes most caregivers. How, they wonder, can they communicate with their care recipient when she has lost the ability to speak and understand what is spoken to her? Furthermore, AD presents many other challenges. The care recipient may not be able to recognize the caregiver or even where she lives. Additionally, care recipients with AD may experience behavioral changes that can aggravate, agitate, and create even more confusion and stress for caregivers. As a result, communicating with someone who has AD can require extraordinary dedication. Caregivers need to realize their old ways of communicating will no longer be effective and must learn new and different techniques.

Many caregivers who struggle with communicating with their care recipients with AD have shared the following:

- "I don't know what to say to my husband. He doesn't even know who I am half the time. Sometimes I wonder if it even matters if I visit with him."
- "My mom doesn't realize she has AD and thinks everything is fine. She is constantly upset with things I say to her."
- "My father now has AD. He was used to always being in charge. He refuses to let me help him with his finances and accuses me of wanting to take his money."
- "My father doesn't understand my mother's AD and says mean things to her. It upsets her and us."
- "My mother rambles and doesn't make sense most of the time. I never know how to respond to her."

These statements represent some of the typical feelings and concerns experienced by many caregivers. They also reflect the lack of understanding about how AD impacts communication. There are many reasons for this.

- People who have AD may have what appear to be odd behaviors and actions. Realize that for them, these actions or behaviors have meaning. For example, a person may take his clothes off in a public place because he is hot, may need to use the restroom, or think it's time for bed. This behavior would normally be out of character, but AD causes impairment to the frontal lobe. This area of the brain helps control impulses and the ability to filter words and thoughts.
- Many people with AD lose their ability to communicate with words. They may use the wrong word or their sentences may be incomplete. For example, they may say they need to rest instead of saying they need to use the restroom. Or they may have "word salad," in which their sentences are said backwards or wrong words are used.
- Some people with AD may have difficulty following conversations and extracting meaning.

Changing the way you communicate with your care recipient is essential to reducing stress for both of you. Remember, AD can present as an "on and off" disease, and your care recipient can change from moment to moment. Be flexible and understand that your care recipient will be more capable of communicating at some times than at other times. You may have to:

- Use one or two words at a time and simplify what you say.
- Use direct statements. For example, you might say, "Now it is time to take a bath," instead of "Would you like to take a bath?"
- Be aware of your body language.
- Point to the subject when trying to communicate without words. For example, you may want to point to your son as you are telling your care recipient about his baseball game.
- You many need to show a picture of what you are trying to communicate.
- Use a positive tone of voice when talking with your care recipient. People with AD seem to be particularly sensitive to how the tone of your voice sounds.
- If your care recipient can still make some decisions, limit the choices to two whenever possible. Making a choice can help her feel that she still has some control in her life.
- Nonverbal communication will become critical to maintaining a relationship. Paying attention to your care recipient's facial expressions or body language can provide clues to his needs or feelings.
- Reminiscing is a wonderful way to connect with your care recipient. Reminiscing helps to tap into memories that are well preserved. I often call these the memories of the heart. Talk with your care recipient about a past memory that he might remember. For example, if your father loved cars, talk with him about the first car he ever owned. Show him pictures of old cars. Long-term memory stays functional for much longer than short-term memory.
- Use the senses. Sensory memory—smells, tastes, touch, and sounds—from the care recipient's past can communicate comfort and a sense of belonging. For example, your mother might have had a flower garden and loved the smell of flowers. Perhaps you could bring a few different roses that offer different smells.
- Don't ask questions. Often the care recipient will not be able to make a decision or answer you. For example, if you ask, "Would you like to . . . ?" a person with AD will often automatically answer no.
- Try not to say the proverbial "Don't you remember . . . ?" When someone has AD, she may not be able to remember, retain, or even understand information. This issue can be quite challenging. It is not unusual for care recipients with these types of memory issues to accuse you of not visiting, even though you were just there.

New Ways to Connect with Care Recipients with AD

Hopefully these points have provided insights and a better understanding of the communication challenges presented when your care recipient has AD. As mindful caregivers, the goal will be to step back and get in touch with how you feel. Then begin to consider the adjustments you will need to make. Journeying through the caregiving experience with someone with AD challenges you to *rethink* how to connect with your care recipient. On the upside, most care recipients have led full, rich lives. They have engaged in activities and experiences that were fulfilling. Even though your care recipient has limited cognitive abilities, it's important to relate to him as a person and not just to the symptoms of the disease. AD does not define the person. It is only one aspect of the person.

Finding Ways to Connect with Joy and Heart

Not all about AD and communication is fraught with challenges. There can be what I call "Alzheimer's defining moments" that can bring joy and smiles to your spirit and soul. These are the moments when something funny or touching may happen, when you learn something new about yourself, or you experience a different side of your care recipient. In my experience, one of the best ways to stay connected to people who have AD is to connect to their hearts and spirit. I believe that the heart remembers, even if the brain doesn't. Think heart, not head. Unfortunately, our culture tends to fixate on our heads. Yet when a care recipient has AD, he will at some point in the disease process lose the ability to process and remember. This can frustrate and sadden you at the same time. You recognize how different your relationship is and how your communication has changed. This can be particularly distressful because we often want relationships to remain stable and stay the same. However, AD teaches you that relationships are in constant flux. My caregiver mantra is to remember "The only control you have is over the changes you choose to make."

People with AD can often thrive and their spirits can be touched in positive ways. There can be new engagement to behold. I have personally and professionally found this to be true. There are several factors that can create these new connections. First, people with AD tend to be more present focused. They live in the moment, and they can teach us about living in the moment. At first this may feel awkward and uncomfortable. Many caregivers are constantly going and doing—so slowing down and not worrying about what you have to do next takes some getting used to. Second, many care recipients with AD may be less inhibited, which can provide more spontaneous affection and laughter. There can be moments that bring joy and even some humor into your relationship. The key, though, is being open to new types of engagements! The following examples illustrate how these new connections can offer humor and grace.

"I Forgot to Die"

There was a time during my mother's AD when she was on a kick, as I called it, about dying. For about a month, she would state she was going to die. She would tell me that I had better say goodbye because she wasn't going to be there the next day. Even some of her caregivers commented about talking with her about dying. I knew she wasn't at the end stages of her disease. In fact, she was still a pretty good picture of health. Yet, I must admit, it rattled me some, and silently I wondered if she knew something I didn't. Well, one day when I was visiting her during this phase of her disease, she said to me, "Nancy, I have to tell you something. You have to promise not to tell anyone." So of course I said, "I promise." Then with a serious voice she said to me, "Nancy, I was supposed to die today, but I forgot!" Taken aback, all I could muster back was, "Mom, I am glad you forgot!" And every time I share that story with others, I still smile.

"The Affair with the President"

Over the years during my spouse support groups, people would repeatedly share how they struggled to handle their spouses' delusions. Delusions can present themselves when people have AD. A delusion is a false belief that remains fixed, even in light of contradictory evidence. In other words, a person with a delusional belief truly believes it is true. This can be very upsetting to caregivers, especially when they have been accused of all sorts of things, from having affairs, to stealing personal effects, to robbing money. I would tell spouses that it would be important to not try to talk them out of their delusions or tell them their delusions were not real. Most caregivers find it hard not to personalize delusions, especially when the beliefs are accusatory. For example, it is not uncommon for a married care recipient to charge his or her spouse of having an affair. Do your best to not personalize what is being said.

Not all delusions are difficult, and I am reminded of a funny story as told by a spouse in one of my group sessions. Audrey was sharing her morning coffee with her husband, Bill, when he turned and proclaimed, "I can't believe you are having an affair with the president of the U.S. How could you do this to me?" Audrey was flabbergasted and could hardly contain her laughter. Yet, remembering the importance of not arguing or refuting the statement, she turned to Bill and said, "Well, at least I pick the best." And then even more shocking to Audrey, Bill quickly retorted back, "You mean second best. I am the best." Audrey turned to Bill and said, "Yes, you sure are!"

The Valentine Rose

Sam came to me because he was struggling with how he would get through Valentine's Day. He had been married to his wife, Rose, for sixty years. Every year, he would buy her a dozen roses and cook dinner. With tears in his eyes, Sam shared that this year, Rose not only didn't know it was Valentine's Day but didn't even recognize him anymore. He was struggling with how to celebrate this day with her. I suggested that Sam allow himself to just be with his feelings. He realized he felt sadness, a little guilt, and even a little anger that his Rose didn't seem to remember him. Then I turned to him and gently said, "It may seem as if Rose does not remember you, but you do remember her. Maybe you should buy a dozen roses as a way to honor your relationship?" After he thought about it for a minute, his whole demeanor changed. He had a big smile on his face and said, "I will buy a dozen roses for my dear Rose and keep them for me!"

These are just a few examples of how caregivers have learned how to be mindful of how they connect with their care recipients so they could be true to their unique situations.

Creative Ways to Connect with Those Who Have AD

> Life is either a daring adventure or nothing.
> —Helen Keller, *The Open Door*

Finding creative ways to connect with your care recipient requires adapting a beginner's mind philosophy. A beginner's mind is a Buddhist term that implies a willingness to stay open to new ways of being or seeing, without judgment. Caregivers need to let go of the mind's rigid boundaries and open their hearts to new ways of being. It may mean allowing yourself to be more playful and silly. And doing so may at first feel like a *daring adventure!* Yet allowing yourself to be creative and less serious can bring unexpected joy to you both.

The following are some new ways to connect with your care recipient:

- Think of the songs that you enjoyed with your care recipient. Maybe it was a theme song from your wedding or a song you both loved to dance to or songs you sang out loud together.
- Consider different ways to celebrate holidays, birthdays, and other important calendar events. You can bring the celebration to your care recipient. And you can consider celebrating them even on a different day, because many people who have dementia don't necessarily realize what day it is anyway. This can take the pressure or guilt off of you for feeling that you have to find a way to celebrate on that day only.

- Create new rituals of being together. For example, one of my new rituals with my mother was creating a "spa day" at her nursing home. Each week, I would reserve a time to take my mother to the beauty salon and wash her hair and face with nice smelling soap.
- Be willing to laugh or be silly *with* your care recipient. Make up songs. Or when you sing familiar songs, make up new words.
- Be willing to be in your care recipient's world. If she thinks she is back in her old home or in a different state, go with it. Shifting to her reality can help lessen your stress and definitely will lessen hers.
- Remember your cherished memories and make it a point of sharing these together. For example, if you both enjoyed singing holiday hymns together, continue to do so.
- Get outside and enjoy nature. Watch the birds or butterflies, enjoy the sunshine, or listen to the sounds of the outdoors.

MINDFUL WAYS TO HAVE A HEALING PRESENCE

Embracing a healing presence requires you to just be in the moment together.

"A healing presence requires being consciously and compassionately in the present moment with another or others."[5] A healing presence allows for each moment to unfold. Prescribing to a healing presence can give caregivers permission to slow down and just be with their care recipients. This is important because in many caregiving situations, the moments change continually. And when care recipients are no longer able to express themselves, learning to just be with them can be a powerful way to connect with one another. As one caregiver shared with me, "I never knew who I would be to my husband or how alert he would at any point in time. I learned how to go with the flow and be with him in the moment." A healing presence affords the opportunity to appreciate what I call "grace moments." These are precious moments that can be missed or taken for granted. For example, I relished watching my mother eat the cheeseburgers I would bring her from the local fast food restaurant. Each bite brought her a sense of delight.

Learning to be a healing presence helps you appreciate all the senses available to be used with your care recipient. It's a wonderful way to connect and to help your care recipient connect to the world around him. It teaches you to pay attention to the ordinary instead of letting it slip away. For example, take Jim, who lives in a nursing home with a beautiful garden. When Jim went outside, he pointed out every bird chirp, making sweet comments about what he thought they were trying to say to us.

The following is an example of how to experience a healing presence.

"The Doctors Hands"

One particularly memorable visit was with a retired physician with AD who was living at the time in a nursing home. He was at the point in his AD where his ability to clearly communicate was becoming more limited. His family hired me to visit him and provide supportive interaction. During my visits, I would read a short section from a book or bring music that we could listen to together. Increasingly, however, he also was sleeping a lot more. On this particular day of my visit, I found him lying on his recliner sound asleep. I thought for a moment about leaving, thinking to myself I would be unable to do much for him that day. Then I stopped and reminded myself about the importance of being a *healing presence*. A healing presence is when you as the caregiver learn to just "be" with the care recipient, often sitting together in silence. In that spirit, I decided to massage his hands and then hold them in mine. I remembered that he had once been able to share how important a physician's hands were in the diagnostic and healing process. "Nancy," he said, "doctors don't touch people enough anymore. When I was learning about medicine, I was taught how powerful a tool my hands would be for diagnosing and healing." Now, sitting with him, I thought about how many people he had touched and healed with his hands. I began to quietly communicate my thoughts to him. I sat with him about a half an hour, just holding his hands and telling him how grateful people were to have been touched by him. Although he seemed to be asleep the whole time, I believe he also heard me and took in my words. It was my turn to have a healing presence.

Last but not least, learning to have a healing presence is one of the best ways for caregivers to tune into themselves. It requires you to move aside the busyness of your life and make room for quiet and calm. It can help you get in touch with how you feel in that moment with your care recipient. It can provide you with a different level of awareness. I recall many times just sitting outside with my mother and watching the butterflies and hummingbirds. It brought me joy and peace and gratefulness for the moment.

THE SACRED ART OF LISTENING FROM THE HEART

> A loving silence often has more power to heal and to connect than the most well-intentioned words.
> —Rachel Naomi Remen, *My Grandfather's Blessings*, 144

In today's world, there is little room for listening. Listening takes time. Unlike what many of us may think, listening is not a passive activity. It actually takes a great deal of effort to listen with intention and concern. Additionally, listening is also a choice. Many of us tend to listen with half an ear and with very little heart. We are more concerned about getting our point across than listening to what the other person is trying to say.

Listening from the heart requires a quieting of the mind. When we listen from the heart, we create a sacred space between ourselves and the people we are listening to. Listening can transform our relationship with our care recipients. Listening with your full attention provides validation to the care recipient. In essence, you are saying to your care recipient that he matters. As a caregiver, you give the gift of your attention.

Listening from the heart also affords positive opportunities for caregivers to get some relief from their own stress. When they allow themselves to listen to their own hearts, they create a stillness within themselves that can help them be more compassionate toward themselves. Many people think that listening is something we do for others. Yet when we listen to ourselves and reflect upon what we are hearing and feeling from within, we have the opportunity to know our heart.

I am reminded of a caregiver, Joan, with whom I worked for several months. She would talk on and on about all she had to do and how she could never get anything done. Just listening to her exhausted me. During the second session, midway through her speed talking, I gently placed my arm on hers and said, "Joan, I want you to stop talking and just sit and be silent for a moment." She looked at me as if I were asking her to fly to the moon. Then she turned and said, "I am afraid of the silence" and began to cry. Many caregivers feel the same way. When caregivers become still, their emotions can come more into focus. In Joan's situation, she got in touch with how her continually doing and talking kept her from feeling. She also realized it prevented her from considering other options and perspectives.

Sam was referred to me because of continual stomach distress, which his doctor believed suspected had to do with the stress of caring for his wife, Marlene. After the second session with Sam, I asked him what about caring for his wife could he not stomach. Interestingly, he answered quite quickly, "I can't stand having to catheterize her." He had been doing so for the last month and it was making him sick. Yet, he was ashamed of saying anything to anyone. He felt like this was "his duty as a husband." He also went on to say that the doctor thought this should not be a big deal. I encouraged him to ask Marlene's doctor to request a home health nurse so that she could catheterize his wife. His doctor agreed. Once Sam was relieved of this duty, his stomach problems went away.

Listening to your heart also helps you to tune into your own inner rhythms. You learn to pay more attention to your body and what it might be telling you. For example, carefully listening to your body may allow you to get more in touch with its signals. You may notice your heart pounding or skipping beats, headaches, backaches, stomach pains, and such. And instead of staying busy and ignoring these signs, perhaps you will reflectively question what your body is saying and take care of yourself first. Too many caregivers I worked with have refused to listen to what their hearts and bodies were telling them. Many of them ended up with heart attacks and other stress-related illnesses. They then became not the caregiver but the one needing care. So be a mindful caregiver, take yourself seriously, and listen to how you are feeling in mind, body, and spirit.

HOW TO SPEND TIME WITH YOUR CARE RECIPIENT AT HOME

> The language of your heart is to be felt not heard.
> —Paula Reeves, *Heart Sense*, 60

In my work with caregivers over the years, I continually heard the same thing from caregivers—they don't know how to spend time with their care recipient, particularly when she has dementia. Many caregivers are able to provide exceptional physical care but tend to either leave out or struggle with how to provide meaningful activities for their care recipient. And in truth, many caregivers are so exhausted by the time they tend to the physical care needs that thinking about tending to the social needs of their care recipient seems impossible. However, finding satisfying ways to be together is important for maintaining your spirit as well as that of your care recipient. Here are some simple ways to engage with one another:

- Consider finding music that both of you enjoy and make a point of playing it several times a day.
- Sing together.
- Dance.
- Exercise together.
- Get out in nature. Sit in your backyard, take a walk in a park, sit by a pond or lake.
- Share food. Foods that bring back memories from childhood can be very soothing. For example, if your care recipient loved the smell of soup or fresh-baked bread, make some. You might cook together, or if that's not possible, have your care recipient close enough to be able to smell the aromas.
- Look through photo albums together.
- Watch TV shows or movies that you both enjoy. For example, one caregiver bought a bunch of DVDs of her mother's favorite shows, such as *I Love Lucy* and *The Golden Girls*. Another caregiver knew his father loved old westerns.
- Read to your care recipient. Find short stories, magazines, or sections from the Bible or other faith-related book. Picture books can be fun to look through as well.
- Give a hand or neck massage.

I hope some of these ideas will bring you and your care recipient some pleasure.

MAKE YOUR VISITS MORE MEANINGFUL

> Mindful caregivers plan their visits, so that they can experience as much ease as possible.

This section is for those of you who have a care recipient in a long-term care facility. Many caregivers struggle with visiting their care recipient when she is in a nursing home or assisted living community. Here are some of their common questions.

- How often should I visit with my care recipient?
- What if my care recipient constantly asks me to take him home?
- How can I make my visits more meaningful for *me*?
- How do I handle my mother when she continually berates me?
- What do I say when he says he hates where he is living?

While each situation is different, there are some helpful hints and ideas that mindful caregivers might want to consider.

- Remember, it is not the length of time or how often that you visit that matters, but the *quality of the visit*.
- Visit when *you* are not rushed, exhausted, or feeling very "visitor *un*friendly." Your care recipients pick up on your energy, or lack thereof. When you are not in a good mood or in a hurry, the visit tends to not feel good for either of you!
- Pick times, if at all possible, to visit when your care recipient will be at his best. This is especially important for those care recipients who have dementia. As the day wears on, many care recipients become more tired and can experience sundowning. Sundowning is the term used to describe elders who have dementia and become more agitated, confused, and disoriented toward the end of the day. Care recipients often have much more difficulty engaging at this time.
- Stay calm and try not to react if your care recipient complains about where he is living. A response might be, "I came to visit with you so we could enjoy our time together. If you are going to complain, then maybe now is not a good time for me to visit." If you leave, it's important to reassure her that you will visit another time. Some caregivers may not find this easy to say or do. Yet, if you want to feel better about your visits, hold onto this tenet. The message you are sending is that you are willing to visit, but it cannot *be only* on your care recipient's terms.

- Find the facility's activities calendar and consider visiting when there are programs that you and your care recipient would enjoy.
- Bring a friend or relative along. This can defuse the stress or sometimes stop your care recipient from complaining or acting out.
- Include another resident in your visit, which can encourage interaction and new connections.
- Consider bringing music that the two of you could listen to together.
- Consider praying together or reading meaningful religious passages.
- Stimulate memories by making and bringing a scrapbook or posterboard collage.
- Use food to connect by bringing something you and your care recipient might enjoy eating.
- Bring a video to watch together.
- Consider massaging your care recipient's shoulders, neck, hands, and feet.
- Bring children or even a pet, as they are great sources of joy and comfort and can shift the focus off of you.
- Give yourself permission to just be with your loved one. You don't have to talk. You can hold hands, go outside, find a nice place inside, lie in bed together, or whatever would comfort you both.
- Create a "circle of support" around your care recipient by asking friends and family to visit every once in a while. You are not the only one who can provide joy and pleasure to your care recipient.

Next, let's look at how to visit with your care recipient during the holidays.

HOLIDAY TIME A MIXED BLESSING

> You can complain because roses have thorns, or you can rejoice because thorns have roses.
> —Ziggy, cited by Fazio et al., *Rethinking Alzheimer's Care*, 113

Over the years, many caregivers have asked me how they should they celebrate the holidays when their care recipient is too frail to come home or has AD. Truthfully, there is no one way. And for some caregivers, this can be a difficult situation as no doubt the holidays can evoke feelings of sadness and joy. Holiday time can already be stressful. Then when you add the care recipient's particular health situation into the mix, you can feel overwhelmed.

There are a number of issues that need to be considered when trying to figure out how to best proceed during the holidays. First, caregivers will want to reflect on how they used to celebrate the holidays. Here are some questions to ask yourself:

- How important were the holidays to the care recipient?
- What role did your care recipient play in during the holiday celebrations?
- Where were the holidays celebrated?
- What was your role and how important are the holidays for you?

Once you answer these questions, you can begin to consider how to best handle the holiday time. Holidays can be overwhelming, and the goal for you is to reduce as much of the stress as you can.

I have found that many caregivers rarely consider their own needs and instead worry more about how their care recipient will fare during the holidays. It's not always easy to separate out what you need with what you believe would be best for your care recipient. The mindful caregiver recognizes that her needs matter too! Holidays can also reinforce how things have changed and bring up feelings of loss. Many caregivers may feel a sense of guilt if they don't celebrate the holidays with their care recipient the way they used to. Yet many care recipients with dementia aren't even aware of when a particular holiday is approaching. Many people in the middle or later stages of AD are not able to follow a calendar or even seasons. As a result, it may not matter if the care recipient celebrates the holiday on the actual holiday day.

I have found that holidays are generally more difficult for caregivers to cope with than for the care recipient. Trying to decide, for example, if Dad should come to our house this year, if we should take Mom out with all of us to dinner, or if we should travel with Mom or Dad to relatives' homes can feel like a tug-of-war on caregiver's hearts. The following are some thoughts to consider that can ease your way:

- Think about the rituals that can still bring both you and your care recipient joy, such as singing holiday songs together, decorating a Christmas tree, or lighting the Chanukah candles.
- Listen to music that brings warm memories of the holidays.
- Share foods that symbolize the holidays.
- Invite young children who can bring holiday cheer like no one else.
- Bring the celebration to your care recipient in the nursing home or assisted living community and remember, it doesn't have to be on the day of the holiday.

If you decide to take your care recipient to either your home or a relative's home, there are some additional considerations. Ask yourself:

- Is the place handicap accessible, inside and outside?
- How ambulatory is your care recipient?

- Will there be too many people, which could overwhelm your care recipient?
- Can your care recipient toilet himself?
- How will your care recipient's behavior impact the holiday celebration?
- Will she want to leave before the event is over, and how will that impact your enjoyment with everyone?

Caregivers cannot only survive during the holidays but also find ways to thrive and enjoy the holidays with a little less stress.

It is my hope that this chapter provided some helpful information and creative ways to have more meaningful engagement with your care recipient. Remember, when you find ways to enjoy your time together, you will have a better opportunity to feel more at ease with your relationship.

NOTES

1. Mary Pipher, *Another Country: Navigating the Emotional Terrain of Our Elders* (New York: Berkley, 1999).

2. Piper, *Another Country*.

3. Ram Dass, *Still Here: Embracing Aging, Changing, and Dying* (New York: Riverhead Books, 2000), 94.

4. Alzheimer's Association, "Alzheimer's Association," www.alz.org/.

5. James E. Miller and Susan C. Cutshall, *The Art of Being a Healing Presence* (Fort Wayne, Indiana: Willowgreen, 2001), 12.

SIX
Navigating the Maze of Professional Resources, Services, and Support

We depend on the civility of other human beings and a vast network of exchanges to live our lives.
                    Mary Catherine Bateson, *Composing a Further Life*, 6

Throughout their journey, caregivers will find themselves in need of all kinds of professional services, resources, and support. There are numerous options out there and it can be challenging, time consuming, and even confusing to figure out what might be the best for you and your care recipient. Unfortunately, I have found that too often caregivers wait until a crisis occurs before they begin to look for help. Then they find themselves in a stressful, urgent situation and are forced to make decisions while emotionally overwhelmed. Mindful caregivers recognize that navigating through this maze requires planning ahead. I hope the information below will help guide you through the maze.

"I'M OVERWHELMED AND DON'T KNOW WHERE TO BEGIN"

Sylvia was ninety years old and living independently. Recently, she had been having some trouble walking and had begun falling. The falls were serious enough that she had been to the ER three times in the past six weeks. Fortunately, Sylvia had not broken anything, but her daughter, Molly, was terrified that the next fall could result in a broken hip. Molly felt frustrated because Sylvia's doctor wasn't offering much help, other than to say that Sylvia should move into a nursing home. Molly was overwhelmed and, at a friend's suggestion, came to see me. She didn't know what to do, who to turn to, or what her options were.

I use this story because it is a very common scenario and one that introduces the content of this chapter. I start with information to help you assess if your care recipient can or should be at home. Next, I describe some of the services that are available to help, both in and out of the home. Then I present information on some of the geriatric professionals, like myself, who can assist you with this journey. Lastly, I end with a description of facilities, should you need to place your care recipient in an assisted living or nursing home. I offer questions to help you assess these professionals and services and make informed decisions. I also list useful online resources, as well as help you evaluate the reliability and authenticity of new sites that are constantly popping up. While I focus primarily on adults with chronic diseases, the information in this chapter can be helpful to all caregiving situations. My hope is to educate, empower, and encourage you.

KEEPING YOUR CARE RECIPIENT AT HOME

How do you determine if you should keep your care recipient at home? There are many different factors to evaluate.

Age and Overall Health

One place to begin is to assess the overall health of your care recipient. Is he healthy enough to remain at home? Does he have a chronic illness that is expected to get worse over time? Can she prepare her meals, take her own shower, do her laundry, and drive to the grocery store, bank, or doctor appointments? Can he keep up the house, inside and out? Does she need assistance? What kind? What financial resources does your care recipient have to pay for services? If resources aren't available, are there family members or significant others who could help out?

Another factor is your care recipient's age. Over the years, I have witnessed numerous "healthy" eighty-year-olds whose health has abruptly and radically changed. Many of these and the following factors need to be considered in the here and now, *and* again if something changes.

Home Environment

If your care recipient is to remain in his home or perhaps live in yours, you need to evaluate the home situation for potential *safety hazards*. When assessing potential safety hazards, I suggest that you go through each room and consider the furniture and other items. Can your care recipient easily navigate around? Are there items that could be removed? Are cords and other obstacles out of the way? Is there sufficient lighting? Can your care recipient safely get in and out of his favorite chair? Can she easily get in and out of her bed or could she fall out of the bed? Are the kitchen and other chairs sturdy, with two arms to facilitate getting in and out of safely? Do the floors have any potential trip hazards? Have throw rugs been removed and carpets secured? Are clothes, dishes, food, and other necessities within easy reach?

The above considerations are important for an elder-friendly and handicap-accessible environment. However, keep in mind that as your care recipient's health declines or a health crisis occurs, it may become critical for the home to be even more accessible. In Sylvia's case, her two-story house made it difficult for her to easily get around; fortunately, there was a bedroom and bathroom on the main floor. Other factors to consider follow. Are there steps in the house that your care recipient will have to navigate? Don't forget about steps that lead into the house or down to another room. Is there at least one bathroom that has a low- or no-threshold walk-in shower? Are there handrails or grab bars in the bathroom and other rooms?

Socialization and Activities

I have found that sometimes caregivers don't give enough credence to the importance of social interaction and activities. If your care recipient is going to live alone, he can become easily isolated, which can lead to depression and other health concerns. Many elders in particular are reticent to admit that they are lonely because they so badly want to remain in their home. Are there neighbors and friends who can still visit with your care recipient? Are there family members who can visit as well?

Transportation

If your care recipient is still driving, it is important to assess her abilities. There are now services that will provide driver safety assessments. Can your care recipient see well both during the day and at night? How is her reaction time? Is he on any medications that could potentially impair his driving, such as pain medications, psychiatric medications, or sleep medications? If she can no longer drive, how will she get her groceries and to her doctor and other appointments? Who will be responsible for setting his transportation up?

Caregiver Needs

Last, but not least, you have to factor in your own health, and physical and emotional resources. Too often caregivers do everything they can to keep their care recipient at home, and do so at their own expense. So step back, be mindful, connect to your heart, and realistically assess the whole situation. Ask yourself if you can realistically take this on and care for yourself and your care recipient.

Let's go back to Sylvia's situation. I met with Sylvia and her daughter, Molly, and made a home assessment. I also created a care plan for them, which included referrals to a variety of professional services. From my home visit, it was clear that her living situation was unsafe. I had Molly decrease the clutter, secure the rugs, and install rails and grab bars. I also suggested Sylvia be evaluated for home rehabilitative services, to see if she might benefit from physical therapy and possibly some aids, such as a walker or three-prong cane. I recommended that Sylvia might go to an elder day program for socialization and some medical oversight. Lastly, I suggested that Molly might want to consider a support group. The next section describes these and other services.

ELDER RESOURCES AND SERVICES

Senior Living and Placement Services

Placement companies are businesses that provide referrals to a variety of services, including home care agencies, residential care homes, retirement communities, assisted living facilities, and nursing homes. Some of these companies are small and run by skilled professionals who are familiar with the local services and facilities. Others are regional or national franchises with consultants who frequently answer the phone out of their home and have never seen the facilities they are referring to. It is very important to understand how some of these companies work and how they charge. Many advertise their consultation services for "free" but will charge the facility or service a fee for listing them in their database. In addition, many receive a referral fee every time they successfully place someone—as much one month's rent or even more. For your average assisted living or nursing home, that can be $4,000 to as high as $12,000 in my experience.

If you choose to use a placement service, you need to find out several different things. If you can, find out if placement services are regulated in your state. For instance, Florida recently changed its assisted living regulations laws and now exempts placement services from the prohibitions on "patient brokering."[1]

What this means in Florida and many other states is that these services are unregulated. Second, find out the qualifications of the consultant. A licensed professional has both an ethical and statutory mandate to disclose third-party fees. Many of these companies are under no obligation to reveal their fee structure.[2]

So before you use them, ask several questions:

- What are your qualifications? Are you licensed by the state?

- Will you conduct a face-to-face assessment of my care recipient?
- What do you charge for your services? Do you get a commission for placing my care recipient?
- Have you ever visited the place you are recommending? When was the last time?
- Why are you recommending the service or facility? What makes it a good match for my care recipient?
- What do you look for in a facility or service? (The answer should include ownership, length of time in business, qualifications of staff, state licensure, and inspection reports.)

Geriatric Care Management

Geriatric care management refers to the process of assessing, planning, and coordinating care for your elder in order to meet his physical and social needs and improve his quality of life. *Geriatric care managers* can come from different professional backgrounds, such as nurses or social workers, or other health fields such as human services or gerontology. Care managers determine the types of services your care recipient needs; facilitate getting and even providing those services; monitor the services, making adjustments as needed; and advocating for you and your care recipient. You should expect that the professional care manager will:

- Provide an *assessment* of your situation and help you determine the "best" placement and/or services for your care recipient. Whenever possible, the care professional should conduct a *face-to-face assessment* of the elder. Meeting with the elder is the absolute best way to ensure an appropriate match of resources and facilities. If the elder lives out of state or too far for the care manager to make a face-to-face assessment, the care manager should determine if there is another professional she could speak with who has currently seen your care recipient.
- Present a written *plan of care* detailing type and rationale for services, the contact information for referrals, and a time line whenever possible.
- Refer you to other *geriatric professionals*, such as geriatric physicians, elder law attorneys, financial managers, and counselors.
- Refer you to appropriate *care environments and services*, including assisted living, nursing homes, home care and home health agencies, hospice care, day programs, rehabilitative centers, and personal care homes.
- Be an *advocate* for you and your care recipient, wherever your care recipient is living—at home, in a nursing home, or in an assisted living community.

- *Communicate* to families and professionals about the needs of your care recipient and report how your care recipient is getting along.
- Ensure the *safety* of your care recipient by evaluating his living environment and identifying potential hazards or problems.
- *Monitor the services* to make sure the plan is being implemented appropriately.
- Provide *case management* services, such as setting up doctor appointments, taking her to doctor appointments, managing the day-to-day affairs of your elder, and regularly checking on your care recipient.
- Help *obtain services and resources* for your care recipient, such as meal programs, transportation services, and financial services.

Geriatric care managers can be incredibly helpful. If you cannot afford one, check with your local Alzheimer's Association, Jewish Family Services, Catholic charities, or other religious institutions. Many organizations provide care management services on a sliding scale.

Adult Day Services and Centers

According to a recent study by Met Life,[3] there are more than 4,600 adult day care centers in the United States. "Adult day services" refers to a structured and supervised program of activities designed to promote the health and well-being of elders, as well as to provide much-needed respite to caregivers. Adult day care centers are open a variety of times. Some centers are open two to three days a week; others operate five or more days a week. And their hours vary as well—from a half day, to open twelve hours a day, to around the clock. Most day care centers provide meaningful activities, meals, and trained support staff. Many day care centers will have a nurse on staff who can monitor vital signs and give medications. Some provide transportation. Additionally, there are day care centers that provide specialized programs for those with chronic diseases such as Parkinson's or Alzheimer's. The cost for adult day care depends upon the sponsor and how many days and hours your care recipient is there. Many day care centers are run and housed in faith-based institutions, although others are nonprofit or for-profit or are privately owned. States differ with regard to their regulations for the operation of adult day care centers. The National Adult Day Services Association (NADSA) offers some useful advice in its Standards and Guidelines for Adult Day Care. This can provide you with the information to help you understand what adult day care can offer in different states.

Counseling

Counseling is a process in which a trained professional talks with another person to help him or her resolve specific problems, gain insight, and cope with situations more effectively. Within the context of caregiving, a trained counselor can offer a variety of help. She can support you as you cope with the unique challenges of dementia, facilitate communication challenges between you and your care recipient, mediate conflicts that might arise within your family, give advice about how best to deal with your situation, and conduct an assessment of your care recipient and give you a plan of care. If you feel an individual counselor might be helpful, I suggest you look for a licensed counselor or social worker with training and expertise in geriatrics, dementia, or family systems. However, if you just need some support and someone that "gets it," then consider a support group. In my practice, I have found that support groups are often exactly what caregivers need.

Support Groups

> "My support group was my lifeline. It was one of the few places in my life I felt understood."
>
> —A caregiver in a spousal support group

Support groups are groups of people with a common interest or concern that meet together on a regular basis. They are or should be led by a trained facilitator. Support groups can offer support, information, resources, and validation. They can be a safe place to share your feelings and concerns with people who are more apt to understand. A common feeling held by many caregivers is that no one can really understand their situation. And to some degree that can be true. Support groups can be very helpful to caregivers because the people in them are facing similar challenges. Support groups also offer a place to ask questions that might be uncomfortable to ask family or friends—such as, how do you handle personal care issues like incontinence, bathing, and mouth care.

There are many types of support groups and it's important for you to find one that fits you. Most are free or charge a minimal fee. Some meet weekly or monthly, some lean more toward being more educational while others are more informal gatherings. Some may be what are called "time limited" or "closed," meaning that once the group has formed, they may meet for a certain length of time or that no one else can join. Other groups are ongoing and open to anyone who wants to attend. It's important to point out that support groups are not and should not be "therapy groups." Well-run support groups usually have a group leader, often a professional or trained leader, who makes sure that the group runs smoothly and that everyone has time to share.

Support groups are not for everyone. However, there are many wonderful benefits to them. If you decide to join a support group, be a mindful caregiver and do your homework.

- Ask who the group leader is, what his background is, and how long he has run the group.
- Find out what sorts of illnesses the members in the group are coping with. For example, is the group made up primarily of people who are caring for someone with Parkinson's disease or Alzheimer's disease?
- Find out the composition of the group. Who is in the group, what are their ages? Is the group composed of mostly of spouses or family/friend caregivers?
- Find out how often the group meets. Does it meet weekly, and will the group only meet for a certain number of sessions?
- How many are in the group? Is there continuity of group members?

Services for elders are an exploding industry. There are many different businesses and individuals offering all sorts of options. I've done my best to describe the various categories of services, but they are not mutually exclusive. Some agencies provide comprehensive services, while others might offer a limited number of services. To further complicate matters, sometimes an individual might provide some of the services and then refer you to an agency for the rest.

HOME HEALTH CARE AND HOME CARE AND AGENCIES

Home Health Care

"Home care" is a term that is used to describe two very different types of care: "*home health care*" and "*home care.*" Home care is nonmedical care that typically focuses on activities of daily living, such as personal care, household chores, and companionship. In contrast, *home health care* is provided by licensed medical professionals and refers to skilled medical care. Home health-care agencies are regulated by state and federal laws. Think of home health care as visiting nurses and other licensed specialists, such as physical, occupational, speech, or respiratory therapists. In most circumstances, these services are often prescribed after a hospitalization. In Sylvia's case, home health care in the form of physical therapy was prescribed by her new geriatric physician as a necessary part of her treatment. With a prescription, these services are generally covered under Medicare, Medicaid, Veterans' Administration benefits, and private insurance, as long as the agency providing the services is Medicare and/or Medicaid certified. But verify your coverage with your individual plan.

Now to really make it confusing, some home health agencies will also provide nonmedical caregiver support or "home care" as well. And some of the skilled medical care can be provided by rehabilitation services or agencies. Let's look at these two groups of services.

Rehabilitation Services

Rehabilitation or rehab services are care and treatment designed to help a person recover from injury, illness, or disease. Sylvia's physical therapy could be provided by a physical therapist employed by home health care agency or by an independent rehab service. The purpose of rehab care is to restore a person's capabilities or help her compensate as much as possible from the problems that have occurred from illness or injury. Rehab care offers many of the same services as home health care, especially with regard to various therapies, such as physical, occupational, respiratory, and speech. Rehab care can be provided in the home, at the person's assisted living or nursing home facility, or in an inpatient rehab facility. With outpatient rehab, the therapist comes to the person and the therapy is generally not as frequent or intense as with inpatient. Additional details on inpatient rehab services are contained in the next chapter.

Home Care

Home care is a very commonly used service that helps caregivers support keeping their care recipient at home. Depending on the state they operate in, they may or may not be licensed. The range of services that home care agencies provide can be quite broad. For example, they can send a *professional caregiver* (as opposed to *family* caregivers) to help your elder with showering, preparing meals, taking medications, or light chores. Perhaps your care recipient just needs some companionship or help with going to and from the grocery store or doctor's office. A reputable home care company will provide professional caregivers who can meet all of these types of nonmedical needs. Depending upon your preferences and resources, agencies can offer professional caregivers on a part-time, hourly, shift, full-time, or live-in basis. As with rehab services, home care professionals can support the care recipient wherever she is, at home, in an assisted living facility, nursing home, or even in a hospital. One last note: Home care services are generally paid out of pocket. Some long-term care insurance policies and government benefits will pay for a limited amount of home care. But as always, check with your individual plan.

Questions You Should Ask

So how do you go about finding an agency? Here are some specific questions to ask.

Agency Credentials

- Is the agency licensed or certified? Almost every state licenses home health-care organizations. However, this is not the case for home care agencies. Medicare and Medicaid will only pay for home care provided by a certified home-care agency. In addition, the Joint Commission is an independent, not-for-profit organization that provides voluntary accreditation for medical facilities, including home care, home health-care agencies, hospices, and nursing homes. Accreditation means they have met certain standards.
- Does the agency provide proof of malpractice and liability insurance?
- Is the agency inspected by an outside organization or the department of health? And if so, what did the last inspection indicate?

Services

- What services does the agency provide?
- Does the agency provide all the services you need?
- When are caregivers available?
- Will a written description of services be provided?
- What procedures does the home care agency have in place to handle emergencies?
- Who provides the assessment of your care recipient? What does the assessment include?
- Does the agency develop a plan of care?
- Do they gather input from the care recipient, her doctor, and family?
- How often will this plan be revised and updated?
- How is the caregiver selected?
- What if you don't like the caregiver or just don't think it's a good match for your care recipient?
- How does the home care agency ensure patient confidentiality?
- Do they work with other geriatric care professionals?
- If so, which professionals and facilities?
- How were they selected?
- Do they have contracts with assisted living, hospice, or nursing homes?

Quality of Services

- How long has the agency been serving this community?
- Does the agency provide references?
- Does the agency assign a supervisor to oversee the quality of care your care recipient receives?
- If so, how often do these individuals make visits?
- How do they work with care recipients who do not want a caregiver in their home?
- What if the caregiver becomes sick on the job or doesn't show up?
- How does the agency track what care was provided to your care recipient?
- Do they provide monthly care reports?
- Who should be called with questions or complaints?
- How does the agency follow-up on and resolve problems?

Costs

- When and how do they bill?
- Is the agency certified to be paid by Medicare and Medicaid?
- Does the agency bill Medicare or insurance companies directly?
- Does the agency furnish written statements explaining the costs?
- Are there payment plan options?
- What are the costs for the different services provided?
- Are there deposits, fees, or any extra costs besides those charged for each service?
- Are you required to use the services for a minimum number of hours per day or per week? Many agencies have a four-hour minimum.
- Is any of the cost covered by insurance or will you have to pay out-of-pocket?
- Are payment expectations in writing?

Agency Staff and Training

- Does the agency require and verify employee references? Do they conduct background checks?
- What are the employee qualifications? Do they have specific job descriptions?
- How does the home care agency select and train its employees?
- Does it protect its workers with written personnel policies, benefits packages, and malpractice insurance?

THE CADRE OF PROFESSIONALS "AT YOUR SERVICE"

Unless someone like you cares a whole awful lot. Nothing is going to get better. It's not.

—Dr. Seuss, *The Lorax*

One of the most challenging aspects of caring for someone with a chronic disease is finding reliable, caring, and supportive professionals. There are many different types of professionals that you may want to consider having on your support team. The descriptions below are very general and meant to give you a sense of what you can typically expect from each type of professional. This is not meant to imply that only that particular professional can provide that service. In addition, I have focused on geriatric professionals—social workers, physicians, and attorneys. Again, that is not to imply that a regular attorney, for instance, won't or can't help you—just that a geriatric professional has extra training working with elders. One final note of caution: Aging has become a big business. Companies, services, and "experts" are popping up left and right. It is important to carefully check out their credentials and experience.

Care professionals can be very helpful to caregivers because they can guide, support, counsel, and advocate for you when you are feeling overwhelmed and stuck. Those who are licensed and trained to provide counseling can be particularly helpful when you have a family conflict or elder resistance. They also can help you cope with your grief and loss, and can provide the same services for your care recipient. Care professionals can be the "go between" person for you and your care recipient's doctor or other health care professionals or elder care specialists. Lastly, because of their vast network, they can help you find resources and services that you may need.

Geriatric Social Worker

A *geriatric clinical social worker* is a professional social worker with expertise working with elders. Most often, the person has a master's degree in social work and additional training and experience in geriatrics, gerontology, or aging. Social workers are licensed by the state and typically provide counseling, assessment, education, and consultation to families and elders. However, there are geriatric social workers who can help with long-term care placement as well. Some also lead support or therapy groups for caregivers or elders.

Neuropsychologist

A *neuropsychologist* is a specialist within the field of psychology who has expertise in assessing a person's cognitive, behavioral, language, and overall functioning. Neuropsychologists, as psychologists, are licensed by the state and should have a PhD from an accredited program. Typically, a neuropsychologist conducts a battery of cognitive tests to determine the strengths and deficits that your care recipient may have. These tests can help you understand if your care recipient has cognitive impairment, and if so, how severe it might be. The results from the testing can also determine what type of supportive services your care recipient may need. Neuropsychological testing can be very helpful when family members are in denial that your care recipient may have cognitive deficits. Additionally, these tests can be extremely helpful when you are determining competency issues.

Geriatric Care Manager

A *geriatric care manager* is a term that represents a cadre of people with diverse backgrounds, trainings, and experiences who help with a range of services for elders. Some care managers have an associate's degree or a bachelor's degree, while others have an advanced degree. Some are trained and licensed in specific disciplines, such as nursing and social work, while others have experience in related fields such as gerontology or human services. Because geriatric care managers as a profession are not licensed and therefore not regulated, it is important for you to ask questions and understand a person's training, experience, and services. You may hear that someone is a "certified" care manager. Several different national organizations offer various certifications for case workers or geriatric care managers. Most certifications require some level of experience, training, and supervision, or a combination thereof, and that the person passes an exam. Just because someone is certified does not make him or her qualified; likewise, just because someone is not certified does not make him or her unqualified.

Questions to Ask Care Professionals

So how do you go about finding a professional to help you? Here are some questions to ask.

- What is your professional training and degree?
- Are you licensed by the state?
- How long have you been working in the field of aging and in what capacity?
- What percentage of your practice is working with older adults and their families?
- What types of cases do you most often work with?
- Are you in private practice or affiliated with an agency or organization?
- Are there other professionals who work with you or for you?

- If yes, who are they and what is their training?
- Who supervises them?
- What services do you provide?
- Are you available in emergencies?
- How do you charge for your services?
- Do you have standard fees for various services?
- Do you accept referral fees?
- Do you accept Medicare or other insurances?
- How do you bill for out-of-pocket expenses such as caregiving supplies, mileage, or other incidental costs?
- What relationships do you have with other geriatric professionals?
- How do you work with them?
- How familiar are you with them? What do your clients tell you about them?

GERIATRIC CLINICIANS

There are many different clinicians with whom you already are or may want to be involved in the care of your elder. Here I describe the most common types of clinicians you are likely to encounter.

Geriatric Physicians

Geriatric physicians or *geriatricians* are doctors who specialize in working with older adults, usually over the age of sixty. Geriatricians have a background in either family practice or internal medicine and then take additional training to become geriatricians. To become board certified in geriatric medicine, a physician must pass a rigorous examination. The goal of geriatric care is to maximize the quality of life of elders. Geriatricians must know how diseases present in older adults and then how to best manage them.

Geriatricians are often referred to as the "gatekeepers" because they oversee the medical care of elder care recipients. Geriatricians make sure that whatever medications your elder care recipient is currently taking are appropriate for her. They are aware of the medications that can cause adverse side effects in the older population. They also are expert at detecting some of the chronic diseases that older adults are more prone to. Geriatricians recognize the importance of working with the older adult's entire health care team as well as with the elder care recipient's caregiver and family. If you cannot find a geriatrician in your area, try to find a physician who has experience working with elders. I highly encourage caregivers to consider finding a geriatrician for your care recipient, especially if she has dementia or other health conditions that require careful management.

Gerontological Nurse Practitioner

A *gerontological nurse practitioner* or GNP is a nurse practitioner with a master's degree from a program specializing in the care of older adults. GNPs are educated to diagnose and manage acute and chronic diseases, and are trained to take a holistic approach to meet the medical and psychosocial needs of older adults. GNPs are licensed nurses and can get board certified in this specialty. How independently the nurse practitioner works depends upon the practice and the state laws.

Geriatric Psychiatrists

Geriatric psychiatrists are medical doctors with training in psychiatry and extra training in geriatric psychiatry. They work with older adults, usually sixty-plus, who have cognitive, psychological, or behavioral challenges that require medical intervention. The primary focus of the geriatric psychiatrists is to help with medication management as it relates to aging, mental, and cognitive health. Therefore geriatric psychiatrists pay particular attention to coexisting medical conditions and are familiar with how medications can help or hurt the elderly. They also understand the importance of working with other professionals who are a part of the care recipient's health care team. As such, they often work in tandem with other treating physicians and health professionals, advising in complex situations.

Geriatric psychiatrists can be an invaluable member of your health care team. Because they are familiar with the cognitive and psychological conditions that elders are more prone to, along with being aware of medication interactions that can occur with older adults, they can truly be lifesavers. They are critical members of your team if you have a care recipient who has had a lifelong history with depression, anxiety, or other mental health issues. In addition, they are extremely helpful when you have a care recipient with dementia who is presenting with multiple issues, from behavioral challenges to depression, paranoia, and so forth. They are best able to tease out dementia from depression and depression from grief. Lastly, they can advise you on how to handle situations that include addictive substances such as alcohol and drugs. In my practice, they have been invaluable assets in helping prevent premature inpatient psych hospitalizations and help manage cognitive behaviors such as paranoia, aggressiveness, agitation, and so on.

Questions to Ask Clinicians

- How long have you practiced?
- Are you board certified? In which specialties?
- What percentage of your practice is focused on elder care?

- What services do you provide?
- What other clinicians work with you and might see my care recipient?
- How will they be involved in my care recipient's care?
- Do you work with other geriatric professionals outside your practice, such as social workers, neuropsychologists, or psychiatrists?
- If my care recipient is referred to specialists, how do you work with them?
- What insurance do you accept?
- How often would you like to see my care recipient?
- If my care recipient has an urgent health problem, how quickly can she be seen?
- How will you communicate with me as the caregiver?
- How do you handle difficult care recipient situations, such as cognitive impairment, alcohol or drug abuse?
- What hospitals, if any, are you associated with?
- If my care recipient needs to be hospitalized, how would that work?
- Do you make visits or do you have a clinician that makes visits to long-term care communities?
- Special questions—if relevant: How do you handle end-of-life matters? What is your philosophy about hospitalization? What circumstances would you need to hospitalize a patient for psychiatric care? Does the hospital have an inpatient unit just for elders?

ELDER LAW ATTORNEYS

Elder law attorneys are lawyers who specialize in and are familiar with the complex and ever-changing laws, policies, and regulations that affect the programs and services used by elders. Caregivers may need to hire elder law attorneys to help them with the legal and financial challenges they may face. The National Academy of Elder Law Attorneys (NAELA) is a professional organization comprised of elder law attorneys, and may be a useful resource to you.

When you work with an elder law attorney, you should expect clear, accurate advice at all times. The attorney should be patient and responsive and should be able to provide you with specific ways she works with her clients. You should always be able to speak with your attorney when you have a question. Keep in mind that elder law attorneys should be familiar with the state laws in which your care recipient resides and can help with:

- Estate planning, including special needs/disability estate planning
- Retirement benefits
- Advanced directives planning

- Long-term care insurance
- Conservatorships and guardianships
- Medicaid planning for long-term care
- Veterans benefits
- Elder abuse and fraud recovery cases
- Nursing home issues and residents' rights

Questions to Ask

- How long have you been in practice?
- Are you a member of the local and national bar association and in good standing? Is there any history of state bar disciplinary action taken against you?
- What areas of elder-law or special needs law do you handle?
- What percentage of your practice is dedicated to elder or special needs law?
- If seeking help with VA or Medicaid qualification, ask how many such cases the attorney has handled and whether any of those clients were denied assistance.
- What types of relationships and networks do you have with other geriatric professionals? For example, are you affiliated with the Alzheimer's Association or other organizations that provide services to your clientele?
- How do you charge for services? Is there a fee for the first consultation?
- How will you work with me and keep me informed?
- Do you have other staff members who will handle my case after the initial meeting, or will there be ongoing contact with you?

BEING A PROACTIVE CAREGIVER

Being prepared is better than wishing you had.

Now that I have covered a range of services and professionals, I want to conclude this chapter with a description of assisted living and nursing homes. Before I do so, however, I can't say enough about the importance of being *proactive*. Being a proactive caregiver requires that you plan ahead as much as possible. You want the opportunity to check out your care options *before* you need them. I hope the following story makes this point.

Howard, Young at Heart

Your father, Howard, is eighty-five years young and has been managing to care for himself fairly well. He still resides in his own home. Out of the

blue, he has a heart attack and ends up in the hospital. After being hospitalized for a week, the hospital tells you your father will be discharged in
a day or two. He is still quite weak, and you are concerned about how he
will be able to manage on his own. You expected him to go to some
intermediate care facility, but you learn he doesn't qualify for rehab. You
can't take him to your two-story home. You check out the assisted living
facility nearby and learn that they have no beds. You start calling other
places and learn how expensive they are. Perhaps your father could go
home and get some help. You struggle with what to do and don't know
where to turn. You naively thought that Medicare covered the costs for
home care or assisted living. To your horror, you learn that Medicare
only covers costs for skilled nursing, not home care and not assisted
living. You father doesn't need skilled nursing. What should you do?

No doubt, this scenario is enough to push any caregiver over the edge.
There are many important reasons to plan ahead and be proactive.

- *Being proactive prevents making quick decisions during a crisis.* Quick
  decisions can be costly both financially and personally. When you
  evaluate facilities ahead of time, you have the opportunity to find
  the best match for your care recipient's needs. If you have to make a
  decision in haste, you may have limited choices and may not find
  the best match. This can create even more stress, as you may need
  to move your care recipient again—which can be personally upsetting and financially costly.
- *It takes time to evaluate potential communities.* When you do your
  homework ahead of time, you can carefully eliminate some places
  and find the ones that best meet your care recipient's needs. Imagine trying to evaluate four facilities in only a few days.
- *Planning ahead often bring more options.* Visiting facilities before your
  care recipient needs one can often open up your options. With time,
  you can visit many different facilities and select the ones that meet
  the needs of your care recipient. Your chances of securing a placement are usually better if the admissions director is familiar with
  your situation. You can also meet the admissions staff and get a
  jump start on filling out the paperwork.
- *Excellent facilities tend to have waiting lists.* In my experience, I have
  found that the best facilities often have waiting lists. Some facilities
  have wait lists of several months to several years. What typically
  happens is you place your care recipient's name on the wait list and
  when an opening comes up, the facility admissions director will
  call you to see if you are interested in moving your care recipient. If
  this applies to a facility you might want, ask how their system
  works and how long it takes to get in.
- *Provides your care recipient with the best opportunity for quality of life.*
  When you evaluate facilities ahead of time, you have a much better

chance of finding the best match for your care recipient. Finding a good match can in turn help ensure quality of life and good care for your care recipient.

Facilities

Assisted Living Communities

Home is where they know you and care about you.

Assisted living facilities, sometimes called ALFs, are housing for elders and people with chronic illnesses. Prior to "assisted living" coming about in the 1980s, there were just nursing homes. Assisted living emerged as an option for people who required less-intense help and skilled care than offered by a nursing home facility but for whom independent living was no longer a possibility. Compared to nursing homes, assisted living environments are usually more like residences and tend to have a healthier population. Assisted living communities are also a way to provide a less-institutionalized environment. Typically ALFs help residents with such personal care tasks as bathing, dressing, grooming, toileting, and meal preparation. These tasks are known as activities of daily living and are sometimes called ADLs.

One important note: You may hear the term "continuing care retirement communities" or CCRCs. CCRCs offer assisted living in addition to other options. A person might enter the CCRC facility with few or no needs and, as such, live independently. As the person ages in place and needs more care, he might move from independent living to assisted living to nursing home care—all at the same location.

Unfortunately, there is not a standard definition of assisted living, and the licensure for such facilities varies state by state. Regulations that govern these facilities are not uniform. Allowable services also vary from state to state. It's very complicated. For instance, one state may not allow assistance with feeding, whereas another state might. Another example is that some states require an assisted living resident to be able to "egress" or leave the building on their own, should there be a fire, for instance. Therefore, it is critical to find out *exactly* what the state requires and regulates, as this affects the care provided. So ask a facility what type of care they can provide.

Also keep in mind that most assisted living facilities have a base price for the lowest level of assistance and charge additionally for each *level of care*. Level of care refers to the type and frequency of assistance your care recipient may need. I have seen assisted living facilities that have three to four levels of care, each with its corresponding charges. For instance, basic assistance with ADLs might be followed by the next level of care. It's tricky to describe, as it depends on what each individual person needs. One person might need incontinence care, while another might need medication management. Others may need hands-on help with bathing, dressing, and grooming. Generally speaking, more time translates into a higher level of care and increased cost.

In addition, many assisted living communities offer what is frequently called "memory care" or dementia care. There is usually a separate price for memory care. If your care recipient might need these services, make sure you understand how they charge and what they provide.

It is important to recognize that assisted living is a very competitive industry. And these assisted living communities want and need your business. Sometimes facilities overpromise the care they can realistically provide to your care recipient. There are many online and print resources available that can help you determine what facility might provide the best care for your care recipient. Some of the most credible websites and helpful books are listed at the end of this chapter. They will help with basic questions regarding care, number of beds, staffing, and available services. Over the years, however, I have come to realize there are some important care issues that separate the good facilities from the mediocre. What follow are some questions and answers to help you evaluate facilities. I suggest you ask the same questions of each ALF and compare the answers.

Q: How does a facility determine the level of care needed for your care recipient?

A: A health professional at the facility should conduct a clinical assessment to assess the level of care needed. Most facilities have a standard form to determine levels of care and it is based upon activities of daily living. Then they should go over the assessment with you. Levels of care translate into time. Essentially, the higher the level of care, the more time required, and the more you pay.

Q: How does the facility manage medications for their care recipients?

A: The facility should ask you for a list of your care recipient's medications, including from whom, for what, and when the medication was prescribed. They should describe procedures that help ensure that your care recipient gets his medications on time and as prescribed. They should also tell you how they handle changes in medications. Every assisted living community has what they call a MAR, which stands for Medication Activities Record. The nursing staff uses the MAR to track your care recipient's current and past medications.

Q: If my care recipient were to have some personal care problems, such has refusing to take a shower or change into clean clothes, how would you handle it?

A: The facility staff should not get defensive or try to convince you that they rarely have care issues. Inevitably, care issues will pop up. For example, your care recipient may become resistant and refuse help with ADLs. Ask for specific examples of how they have handled an emotional issue, such as depression, or a behavioral issue, such as resisting a shower. The staff should be able to describe how they have handled the situation with other residents. Their response should instill confidence that they are dedicated to addressing the issue quickly, safely, and compassionately.

Q: How do you determine if a resident requires hospital care? And how often do your residents go to the ER and for what reasons?

A: There should be a written protocol to address medical emergencies. Ask what that protocol is. The facility should be able to provide examples of when a resident would need to go to the ER and when he would not. In addition, the facility should describe the skills and training of the staff members who assess the emergency, and the hours they are available. Most reputable facilities have a nurse at least during the day, and some facilities have someone available twenty-four/seven. And in these facilities, elders are not sent to the ER as frequently. If your care recipient is being sent to the ER more than two times in a month, the facility should discuss with you why this is happening and help come up with a plan to keep your care recipient out of the hospital. In some cases, continual hospital visits might mean that the care facility is no longer the appropriate place for your care recipient.

Q: What are the circumstances in which you could no longer care for my care recipient? And how is this communicated?

A: The facility should be able to define exactly what the state requirements are and give specific reasons and under what circumstances they *could not* provide safe and appropriate care. Depending on the state, there are different reasons for "discharge." For example, some facilities will discharge your care recipient if he can't transfer himself from his bed to a chair without help or if he keeps falling. Typically, you get a thirty-day notice that the facility will no longer be able to provide care. Another example is when your care recipient becomes combative toward staff or other residents. In this example, the discharge may happen immediately. Ask to see the resident contract, as there should be a clause about what determines termination of the contract.

Q: Are there circumstances in which I would be required to hire additional caregiver help for my care recipient?

A: A facility should be able to describe the circumstances in which this would be required. One of the most common situations is that the facility can no longer keep your family member safe. One example would be that your care recipient is able to wander off premises because the facility is not secured. You may be required to hire an additional caregiver just for your care recipient. Another example might be that your care recipient falls frequently. The facility may require a caregiver to be with your care recipient in order to try to prevent the falls. Keep in mind that if you don't want to hire an additional caregiver, or can't afford to, the facility can discharge your care recipient.

Q: When would my care recipient need a memory care unit instead of regular assisted living?

A: I often share with caregivers that there are usually three major reasons your care recipient may require memory care, and these are *safety*, *structure*, and *behaviors*. If your care recipient is not able to recognize situations in which he might be placing himself at risk (can't discriminate between apple juice and a cleaning solution or may allow a stranger in the house) or when you can no longer keep her safe (may wander out of the house), these would be safety issues. Structure issues involve organizational skills and the ability to motivate oneself to accomplish the various tasks and activities required each day (can't make decisions, can't initiate activities, or requires supervision during activities). Behavior issues involve the inappropriate actions your care recipient may do (taking clothes off in front of people, walking outside without clothes on, or pinching or hitting someone because he is confused).These three issues generally require a more structured and secure environment where there also are more staff members and activities that are specifically geared for people with cognitive impairment.

Q: What do you provide in your memory care program?

A: A quality memory care program should offer an environment that is smaller, self-contained, and provides a feeling of warmth, comfort, and safety. The environment should have dedicated, caring staff members who have all been trained to work with people with dementia. Activities should be geared to those with cognitive impairment. In my experience, meaningful, appropriate activities and socialization seem to help people retain their cognitive skills a bit longer and can lessen depression, anxiety, and other behavioral issues.

Q: How often do you train your staff, and do you offer specialized training? If so, what are the topics?

A: Staff members should receive regular, ongoing training as required by the state. However, I have found that the better facilities offer staff additional training to help them provide good care. One such example is training staff on how to handle emotional and behavioral issues.

Now that I have shared some important questions to ask assisted living facilities, let's move onto the nursing home arena.

Nursing Homes and Custodial vs. Skilled Nursing Care

> The basic human need to continue "being who I am" is perhaps the most important need of anyone living in a nursing home.
> —Burger et al., *Nursing Homes*, 11

Most caregivers will do whatever it takes to keep their care recipient out of a nursing home, sometimes to the detriment of their own health. In my experience, most caregivers have exhausted all resources, personal and sometimes financial, by the time they admit their care recipient into a nursing home. On the flip side, I have had some caregivers share that their nursing home experience was a "lifesaver" for them and their care recipient. They don't know what they would have done without it. Their care recipient was at the end stages of his disease and needed more nursing care than what could have been provided at home or in an assisted living facility.

Nursing homes provide the highest level of medical care outside of a hospital. Most people in nursing homes have serious medical conditions, are at the end stage of their disease, or are people with traumatic injuries that require twenty-four/seven care. All nursing homes provide *custodial care*. Custodial care refers to hands-on care related to activities of daily living, such as feeding, bathing, and dressing. Most, but not all, nursing homes provide *skilled nursing care*. Skilled nursing care refers to the range of services provided by registered nurses and other professionals. This distinction is important. If your care recipient needs certain procedures or specialized medical care, such as intravenous injections, catheter insertions, or complicated medication management, then she needs to be in a skilled nursing facility.

All nursing homes have a medical director who supervises and manages the care, along with nurses and other health professionals such as registered dieticians, physical therapists, occupational therapists, and respiratory therapists. Collectively, the health care team provides whatever care and therapy your care recipient might require. Lastly, nursing homes can offer specialized equipment, such as "geri-chairs," a type of recliner and hospital beds that are not allowed in most assisted living facilities. These types of equipment can be extremely helpful because they offer ways to keep your care recipient safe and comfortable.

Below are some questions for you to ask in order to weed out the good facilities from the mediocre. I suggest you ask the same questions in each facility you visit so you can obtain a comparison of how each facility answers these critical questions. After each question, there are answers that represent a reasonable response.

What are the critical factors I should I look for in a nursing home? Here are key characteristics and questions to ask when touring a facility.

- *Overall Environment*: How does the environment feel to you? Despite the fact that there are many elder individuals who are quite ill in nursing homes, the environment can still feel upbeat and positive. Residents should be engaged with staff. There should be a sense of a "caring spirit" in the building.
- *Facility*: Is the facility clutter free, and does it look and smell clean? Realize that most residents in nursing homes are incontinent so occasionally you will have those types of smells in the hallway. However, if it reeks of those smells, there may be a serious problem with cleanliness of the facility.

- *Staff*: Does the staff seem to know the residents? Is the staff compassionate and caring? How do they handle staff absences? Observe how staff members interact with the residents, and how the residents respond to them. A critical factor is the facility's ability to provide continuity of care and retain staff. In the best nursing homes, staff retention is high. And they have a good system to cover staff shortages and call-outs with internal staff versus hiring outside temporary staff who won't know the residents.
- *Residents*: Are the residents comfortable? For example, do they look like they have been properly fitted in the wheelchair? Do you notice that those elders who are seated in geri-chairs have cushions or other protection to prevent skin tears or pressure sores? Are the elders well groomed and dressed appropriately? For example, are their clothes clean? Does their hair look clean and combed or brushed?
- *Activities*: Are residents out of their rooms and in activities? Observe an activity and see if it seems appropriate and not childish. How involved are the residents and staff with one another during the activity? Do they seem to be having fun or enjoying themselves?
- In addition, Medicare provides a comprehensive checklist, available at www.medicare.gov/nursing/checklist.pdf.[4]

Strong-Willed Sylvia

Molly was very pleased with the care plan we created for Sylvia. Her house was much safer and the physical therapy was helping, but the therapist recommended that Sylvia use a walker or cane because he was still concerned about her balance. Sylvia was a little stubborn and proud. She went to her weekly bridge game at her friend's house in a nearby town and left her walker at home. While going up the stairs, she tripped, fell, and broke her hip. The next chapter will provide information about how to advocate and partner with the staff when your care recipient enters into a care facility. This was the case with Sylvia. She ended up in the hospital, then went into an inpatient rehab facility; much to both Molly's and Sylvia's strong convictions to have Sylvia remain in her home, she had to go into a nursing home.

NOTES

1. Diane C. Lade, "Services Eager to Show Seniors the Way to a Home," *Sun Sentinel*, November 18, 2012.

2. David Spiegel, "The Questionable Lure of Free Long-Term Care Placement Services," *Kaiser Health News*, July 28, 2011, www.kaiserhealthnews.org/Columns/2011/July/072811spiegel.aspx.

3. MetLife, "Adult Day Services: Providing Support to Individuals and their Family Caregivers," MetLife, 2010; available at www.metlife.com/mmi/research/adult-day-services.html#findings.

4. Medicare.gov, "The Nursing Home Checklist," http://www.medicare.gov/nursing/checklist.pdf.

SEVEN

Being a Partner and Advocate in Care

When spider webs unite they can tie up a lion.
—Ethiopa African proverb, *A Tiny Treasure of African Proverbs*

Caring for another person is difficult enough. In addition to all the changes that take place with your care recipient's health, you also have to deal with many new care environments and professionals. There is no doubt that navigating through the complicated health care system can cause great stress and unending worry. In my practice, many caregivers have expressed how helpless and powerless they have felt when trying to advocate for their care recipients when their care recipient is in the hospital, an assisted living community, or a nursing home. *Advocacy* refers to the actions you undertake in support of your care recipient. There are many opportunities and situations in which you can proactively and positively advocate for your care recipient. Advocacy and partnering go hand in hand. *Being a partner in care* is a term I have created. It means learning to work together with the care staff so there can be best outcomes for everyone—your care recipient, you, and the facility. Being a partner in care can also help you take better care of yourself.

This chapter aims to empower you, so you can feel less intimidated by this aspect of the caregiving journey. It begins with a discussion on how to advocate for your care recipient when she is in the hospital or rehab center. Then the focus shifts to helping you advocate and become a partner in care when your care recipient enters a long-term care facility, whether in an assisted living community or a nursing home. These are the most common settings you are most likely to encounter.

WHAT YOU NEED TO KNOW ABOUT HOSPITAL CARE

Hospitals are not the most "hospitable places" for elders.

Why start with the hospital setting? Sylvia's story is a great example. As you read in chapter 6, Sylvia's daughter thought everything was going along as well as could be expected. Then what frequently happens, and totally catches people by surprise, is a crisis occurs, and boom! Your parent lands in the hospital. Unfortunately, it is also too common for elders to fall, fracture or break their hip, and then need surgery. Other common crises include a stroke, a heart attack, or sudden change in the disease. And more times than not, the hospitalization triggers a whole series of events—new and more skilled care requirements, placement into assisted living or a nursing home, or even hospice. When your care recipient has an advocate, however, the outcome can be much improved.

In my practice, I have had many caregivers express that the hospital encounter was one of the worst experiences they have ever had to face. To begin with, many elders find hospital environments frightening and overwhelming—which can exacerbate confusion and agitation in many older adults. The hospital can be an unfamiliar environment with unfamiliar people doing unfamiliar things. When an elder is hospitalized, it is not uncommon to have his or her many medications changed, removed, or supplemented—which can cause additional problems. Furthermore, communicating with elders can be difficult if they have poor eyesight, hearing loss, or dementia. Elders with dementia or hearing loss can easily misunderstand or misinterpret what is being said or done to them. And it can be difficult for them to share whether they are in pain. Constant medical monitoring and invasive tests and procedures can be upsetting for any of us. When an elder has some cognitive impairment, it can be even scarier. Your care recipient may resist treatments, pull out tubes, or even try to leave. Anesthesia, if needed for your care recipient, can cause dementia-like symptoms, such as confusion, agitation, memory loss, and sometimes even hallucinations. Keeping all this in mind is extremely important to being prepared for your hospital experience.

ADVOCATING IN THE EMERGENCY ROOM

In my experience, most of my elders enter into a new phase of their journey by way of the emergency room, or ER. Being aware of what you may encounter in the ER can ease the trip.

ER Admissions

Emergency rooms or ERs are often busy, noisy, crowded places, filled with people experiencing a health crisis. As an advocate, your first goal is to figure out how to keep your care recipient comfortable and calm while you wait to be seen. When a care recipient has dementia, a long wait and overstimulating environment can cause agitation and other behavioral challenges. Whenever possible, tell the admissions staff that your care recipient has dementia and ask if she could be placed in a quiet room until she is seen by a doctor. They may or may not be able to accommodate your request, but it's worth a try. If they can find a separate room, it can help minimize your care recipient's angst and yours as well.

Seeing the ER Doctor

So how long will you wait in the ER? Your wait time depends on many different factors, including the capacity of your particular hospital, your care recipient's health, and how many others are also waiting to be seen. Most ERs use what is called "triage," which means that the most seriously ill or injured patients are seen first. If there are a lot of critically ill people in the ER, your wait time could be very long if your care recipient does not have a life-threatening condition. In Sylvia's case, her hip fracture was not life threatening, but she was in significant pain, and she arrived at the ER in an ambulance. Because of that, she was seen quickly.

Once the ER doctor sees your care recipient, she will examine him and determine the next steps. If tests or procedures are needed, you may have to wait some more. Once the doctor assesses your care recipient's situation, she will then determine whether he will need to be hospitalized, needs short-term care, or can go home. If your care recipient can go back home, ask for the discharge papers and make sure you understand how best to care for your care recipient. Find out whether he will need prescriptions or special instructions about food, activity, or medical devices.

If your care recipient needs to remain in the hospital, find out if your care recipient will be placed in *observation* or be *admitted* to the hospital. This is extremely important! Each is quite different and has major implications for out-of-pocket expenses. Let me explain.

Observation

Observation means that your care recipient will be placed in a section of the hospital to be watched or "observed." Think of it as a halfway point between the ER and full inpatient hospitalization. He will receive care and then be discharged when the hospital care team deems it safe for him to go home. However, he is also considered an "outpatient," meaning he was *not admitted* to the hospital. This has major implications! Keep in mind that patients can be kept in observation for days. So it's very understandable to think your care recipient is "hospitalized." Make sure you confirm his status.

How can observation cause difficulties for you and your care recipient? First, Medicare and many other insurance plans reimburse differently for observation versus hospitalization. So your out-of-pocket expenses could be significantly higher. Second, if the ER recommends that your care recipient go to a rehabilitative facility, Medicare and many other insurance plans *will not* cover it. Many plans require a prior hospitalization; observation does not quality as hospitalization. I have had clients who incurred thousands of dollars of out-of-pocket expenses because their elder was not admitted to the hospital. Since their care recipient was "at the hospital," they just assumed—incorrectly and very costly. Third, observation may not be in the best interests of your care recipient. Recent changes in Medicare have created a negative side effect. In trying to decrease medically unnecessary hospitalizations, rein in costs, and reduce fraud, Medicare now penalizes hospitals financially if patients are discharged and then readmitted in less than thirty days. If your care recipient is in observation, gets discharged, but then needs hospitalization within thirty days, the hospital would not get fined because your care recipient hadn't originally been admitted to the hospital. In fact, a recent study found that after these changes in Medicare, patients kept under observation had increased 25 percent, and they were being kept there for as long as seventy-two hours.[1]

Admissions

Admittance means that your care recipient will be admitted to the hospital for the purpose of receiving inpatient medical care. The ER physician makes that decision. Your care recipient will be admitted under a certain level of care, may be upgraded or downgraded from that level of care, and may also be moved to a particular hospital unit or floor depending on his medical condition. Additionally, your care recipient's *admission status* can change from day to day. And as his advocate, you will need to stay on top of his admission status. Lastly, it's important to know that your care recipient will usually be assigned a *case manager*. A case manager oversees your care recipient's case, coordinates with the health care team, and helps plan for discharge. This individual also helps you monitor your care recipient's status and progress. Thus it will be essential that you get the name and phone number of the case manager and communicate regularly. Armed with this information, let's now examine what you need to know when advocating for your care recipient when she is in the hospital.

ADVOCATING IN THE HOSPITAL

One of the most critical and immediate needs in any hospitalization is to establish a single *point of contact* who will be responsible for communication. In my experience, too many cooks makes for a bad recipe. In other words, when multiple family members are interacting with hospital staff, information can get lost and miscommunication can occur. This can cause enormous stress and frustration. It's best that the care recipient designate one person, and I recommend that it be the POA for health care whenever possible. However, if you don't have a POA for health care, the "point of contact" will need written permission in order to talk with the hospital staff.

Once you have established your point of contact, the following tips can help you advocate for the best care. You will want to stay involved and understand the prescribed treatments and therapies. Here's how:

- *Get to know the charge nurse.* The charge nurse is the person responsible for the care of your care recipient. If possible, introduce yourself to the charge nurses on each shift that will be providing care to your care recipient.
- *Remember you have the right to ask questions.* If you feel you don't understand why a treatment or procedure was ordered, you can ask to know why.
- *Make sure you find out what medications* your care recipient is being given while in the hospital (as well as before and after discharge).
- *Realize you have the right to request to see your care recipient's medical record at any time.*

If you are having any problems or concerns:

- *Talk to your care recipient's primary care doctor.* He may be able to intercede for you if you are having any difficulties understanding what is going on or why.
- *Ask to speak with the supervisor of the unit* if you are having difficulty talking with either the doctor or the charge nurse. In most situations, the unit supervisor can help connect you with the professional who can provide the information you need.
- *Consider hiring* a clinical geriatric social worker or geriatric care manager to help oversee the care or intervene if needed.
- *Consider contacting the hospital ombudsman* if you still have concerns. The hospital ombudsman is a professional specifically designated as a patient advocate and one who can help resolve issues.

Getting Ready for Discharge

As soon as it is reasonable, find out when your care recipient will be discharged or released from the hospital. While this seems like it should be a relatively straightforward process, many times it is not. The doctors, nurses, and case manager work together to determine how long your care recipient needs to be in the hospital. With older adults, however, there are issues that can complicate determining the length of the hospital stay. Elders tend to have more complex medical issues to start. Their admitting diagnosis can change during the time they are admitted into the hospital, which then can alter the length of stay. Sometimes cognitive behavioral issues can make it more difficult to provide treatments to elders, which can also lengthen the stay and delay discharge. The hospital and the health care team also have to follow guidelines set forth by the Centers for Medicare in order to get reimbursement for the hospital stay. These guidelines specify the length of stay and standard treatments for each diagnosis. What this means is that your care recipient could be discharged earlier than you would expect. Too often caregivers have called me in a panic because their care recipient is going to be discharged in a day or two. Since they haven't planned ahead, they then are scrambling to figure out the next steps.

Discharge

The discharge process of your care recipient's hospital stay is a critical aspect of ensuring the best possible recovery. Yet, for some, it can be the most exacerbating aspect of the hospital stay. To ensure the best possible outcomes, let the case manager know that you expect to be told as soon as possible when your care recipient will be discharged. And stay on top of that date. Ask the case manager whether your care recipient will be discharged back home or to a facility so you can make appropriate plans for the next transition.

There may be a number of reasons that your care recipient may not be able to go home. Your care recipient may be too weak or frail and requires skilled care services such as physical, occupational, or speech therapy, or medical treatments that need skilled medical care. Or, your care recipient's home may not be safe or accessible for him. It is also possible that your care recipient's cognitive health may have declined to such an extent that she cannot safely live by herself without help. If your care recipient is going home, review the previous chapters and what is needed to make sure the home environment is safe. If your care recipient *cannot go home*, find out what type of care the doctor is recommending. It could be rehab care, assisted living care, nursing home care, or hospice care. If you have been proactive and researched facilities, you can provide those names to the case manager. If you don't have recommendations, the discharge professional will give you a list of facilities. If your care recipient is going to be transferred to a facility, your next challenge is trying to ensure a comfortable and safe transfer. In Sylvia's situation, her home was no longer an option and her doctor recommended rehab. Fortunately for Molly, the best rehab center had a bed—but I impressed upon her the importance of finding a long-term care facility for her mother, as I suspected Sylvia would at some point be making that transition.

TRANSITIONING YOUR CARE RECIPIENT INTO A FACILITY

It seems to me that one is forced to make inner and outer readjustments all one's life. The process never ends.
— Eleanor Roosevelt, *You Learn by Living*, 78

Transitioning your care recipient into rehab or a long-term care facility can be fraught with overwhelming details, paperwork, and emotional angst. To help ease your way, there are some important steps to be mindful of when transitioning your care recipient. I have called these the "Ready," "Get Set," and "Go" phases.

Ready

There are many different aspects of the transition in need of consideration. This is what I call the get "ready" phase. The ready phase is the behind-the-scenes work that is needed. Hopefully you have checked out the facility ahead of time. If not, you have the right to check out the facility before your care recipient is discharged. The facility has to meet the needs of your care recipient. Next, make sure the case manager finds out *exactly what discharge paperwork* is needed from the receiving facility. For example, there may be specific forms that the hospital physician or other hospital staff members will need to fill out. This is an extremely critical aspect of the transitioning process and can facilitate your care recipient being properly admitted to and taken care of at the next facility. The information on those forms helps staff in the receiving facility provide the next level of care. It is crucial that you stay on top of this process, and it may take several phone calls back and forth between the hospital and receiving facility.

Get Set

The "get set" phase helps to ensure as safe a transition as possible. The following are some basic questions about some important issues:

- *Required Forms*: If your care recipient is being admitted to a *nursing home under Medicaid*, there are particular forms that the doctor needs to fill out. They are the DMA6 and Level One forms. Usually, the nursing home admissions director will fax these forms over to the hospital for the discharge hospital doctor to fill out and send back.
- *Transportation*: Have you determined how your care recipient will be transported to the receiving facility? Can he be transported by car or will he need an ambulance or nonemergency transport? If an ambulance is needed, most insurance plans only pay if a doctor has written an order. If not, you may need to consider nonemergency

transportation that can accommodate wheelchairs or stretchers. Find out if you will have to pay for this service out of pocket.

- *Ambulation Devices*: Will your care recipient now require a walker, wheelchair, or cane?

    1. If your care recipient is using an ambulation device in the hospital, most likely you will not be able to take that device with you.
    2. Make sure you find out exactly what she will need. Ask the facility who will be ordering it whether it will be available when your care recipient arrives.

- *Medications*: How will your care recipient's prescription records and actual medications get transferred to the receiving facility? It's so important to make sure your care recipient gets the medications he needs. Unfortunately, medication errors are fairly prevalent when someone is being transferred to another facility. This issue requires your upmost diligence.
- *Specialized Care*: Are there any ongoing medical issues that need special care? This could include catheters, wound care, or oxygen that will require special care or skilled nursing services. Make sure that there are clear instructions and that the facility has appropriate professionals who will be available to provide these services.
- *Personal Items*: Are there personal items that will help your care recipient feel more comfortable? What items you can bring will depend upon the facility. This could include simple items such as pictures or a favorite pillow. For more permanent placements, this might include electronics or furniture.

Go

The "go" phase is when you begin to advocate and be a partner in care for your care recipient. This is the time in which your care recipient moves into a facility, whether it's a rehabilitation (rehab) center, an assisted living facility, a nursing home, or hospice. Rehab following a hospitalization is commonly used to continue the care for a variety of illnesses and conditions. That makes it a frequent "stopover" before someone enters a long-term care facility. But most of my suggestions for the "go" phase apply to long-term placement. Before we go there, let me briefly discuss rehab.

REHABILITATION CENTERS

As was mentioned in the previous chapter, rehab care is designed to help a person recover or improve his or her health after an injury, surgery, or illness. Inpatient rehab care can be provided in a hospital, a freestanding rehab facility, or in a nursing home with a specialized rehab section. If your care recipient is going to be transferred to an inpatient rehab facility, it is imperative that you make sure your care recipient has met the requirements needed for reimbursement for the rehab care. Medicare and many other health insurance plans will only pay for rehab if your care recipient has had a three-night hospital stay with inpatient status. Rehabilitative care can be thousands of dollars, so it is critical that you make sure insurance will cover the costs.

Rehab care typically lasts between a few weeks to a few months but greatly depends upon the health issue and whether your care recipient can improve. This is a critical aspect of rehab care; the person must be making progress with the prescribed treatment. If the person is not making progress or has made as much progress as is possible, he or she will no longer qualify for rehab care and the care recipient will be discharged. This is very important, as you may be forced to find the next placement for him in a very short time period.

The number of days of needed and authorized rehab care depends on many factors—the diagnosis, the severity of the problem, and the possibility of improving, among them. Medicare and many private insurance plans limit the number of days they will reimburse for rehab. In an approved facility, Medicare covers twenty days of rehab care at 100 percent of costs. If your care recipient needs additional rehab care, he must qualify. Once qualified, Medicare will pay up to 100 days per calendar year at 80 percent of costs. The remaining 20 percent of costs may be covered under a secondary insurance plan if your care recipient has such a policy. If you are utilizing a health plan other than Medicare, investigate what your care recipient's plan will cover with regard to rehab care.

Once your care recipient is in rehab, get to know the staff. Usually these professionals consist of physical therapists (PTs), occupational therapists (OTs), speech therapists (STs), respiratory therapists (RTs), and social workers. One or more of these individuals will work with your care recipient and determine how long she qualifies for rehab care. Generally, a rehab social worker will be the professional to keep you updated on your care recipient's progress. And it is critical to understand that your care recipient has to continue to make progress in order to stay in the rehab center. Once the rehab professionals determine she is no longer able to make progress or she has reached a plateau in her therapy, the care recipient will be discharged. And unlike the hospital setting, the rehab professionals will set up a discharge meeting to discuss next steps when your care recipient is close to discharge. In most situations, once your care recipient has completed his rehab services, he will be transitioned home or to a long-term care facility, either an assisted living facility or a nursing home. As was the case for Sylvia, she completed six weeks in rehab and then needed assisted living.

BECOMING A PARTNER IN CARE

The go phase involves learning to be a partner in care. And being a *"partner in care"* is one of the least talked-about and yet most essential aspects of tending to your care recipient in a long-term care facility. When your care recipient is placed into a long-term care facility, his day-to-day management transfers to the facility staff. Your role shifts and you now become a *secondary caregiver*. This requires learning how to *partner* or find ways to positively work together with the staff members. (Appendix A contains important information that you should compile about your care recipient and share with the facility.) The following is an example of how to become a partner in care.

"Ansell Adams in Disguise?"

Ever since Melanie moved into an assisted living community, she had become extremely depressed. Her children came in for a consult to discuss how to get their mother more engaged. They told me what a happy person their mother used to be and how much she enjoyed people. In fact, Melanie had been active in several clubs and organizations, and was an avid photographer who traveled all over the world. Since her move, however, Melanie's children would find her in bed sleeping or sitting in her room by herself. They had talked with the activities director about their concerns and asked that she be escorted to activities. Although the staff tried all sorts of different approaches to try to engage her, she refused to attend activities. The staff felt frustrated and her family continued to feel disappointed and upset.

I suggested to them that they consider becoming a partner in care and help Melanie become more involved in activities. I recommended they take advantage of her photography hobby and bring in some of her photos. Perhaps they could even ask the activities director to hold a "showing" of her work. They set up a meeting with the activities director and she loved the idea. The event was a huge success! And with this one out-of-the-box idea, a bunch of doors opened up for Melanie. First off, the caregivers and other staff were blown away by her talent. They saw a side of Melanie they hadn't known before. Second, Melanie became more talkative and engaged. Residents and families would compliment her on her amazing pictures. In fact, Melanie became known in that community as the "female Ansell Adams." Her family was thrilled. This is an example of partnering in care.

Not every situation will turn out as positively as Melanie's, but there are many different things you can do to become a partner in care. My hope is that if you do most of these actions, you and your care recipient will find more ease.

- *Get to Know Staff:* Introduce yourself to all your care recipient's nurses and caregivers. This is particularly important so that the staff members are aware that your care recipient has an advocate in her life. In addition, ask about them—where they are from, if they have children, or what they enjoy doing. Caregivers sometimes feel that families don't care about them.

- *Be Available for Questions:* Let the staff know that you are available for any questions or concerns they might have about your care recipient. Without permission, some caregivers may be intimated or afraid to ask you questions.

- *Share Helpful Tips:* Make sure you offer staff the tips you found successful in helping with your care recipient. For example, if there was a certain way to bathe or provide grooming to your care recipient that was more comfortable for him, make sure you explain that to the staff. Or if your care recipient isn't an early morning person, ask if it is possible to wake her up last. Of course, these need to be reasonable and you will need to check with the staff to make sure they are doable. Remember, partnering with the staff helps to ensure the best quality of life and care for your care recipient. It also demonstrates that you appreciate them and recognize the importance of their jobs.

- *Write It Down*: Consider writing down your tips for all shifts. I have found it helpful to use an index card that lists the tips and give this information to the charge nurse. She can then write it down on your care recipient's chart.

- *Suggest and Join in Activities:* Let the staff know what activities your care recipient would most enjoy. In the first few months of the placement, you may need to ask them if your care recipient has been participating in activities. In some situations, it might be helpful to participate with your care recipient.

- *Personalize It:* Make sure you have plenty of pictures and memorabilia in your care recipient's room. It helps the staff get a feel for your care recipient and shows them that family members care and want the room to be comfortable and familiar. In addition, share something new about your care recipient when you come to visit. Talk to the nursing and activities staff and tell them a quick story or show them pictures of your care recipient during different times in her life.

- *Compliment Staff*: Find ways to compliment the staff when you see them doing something good or kind. People are always quick to complain, but the opposite is unfortunately not true. You would be amazed at how little they hear good things from their supervisors or from caregivers or family members.

- *Choose Your Battles*: Be aware of what is most important for your care recipient. That may be different from what is important to you, so learn to "choose your battles!" For example, you might come to visit and find your care recipient with fresh food stains on his clothes. It's important to find out *why* your care recipient wasn't changed into clean clothes. Perhaps it just happened, they were short-staffed, or your care recipient was so agitated that they were unable to change his clothes. Just remember: Before you become too upset, employ mindfulness. Pause for a moment, take a deep breath, and connect to your heart. Ask the following: "Do I need more information before I get upset?" "Is this a situation in which I need to choose my battles?"

THE UNSUNG HEROES: THE CARE STAFF

Another important aspect of being a partner in care is getting to know the care staff and all they do. Many of these staff members can become *like family* to you and your care recipient. It's important to realize that most of the staff members who work for the long-term choose this work out of their desire to help and be of service to others. Many would say they "were called to do this work." Their jobs are difficult and demanding, particularly for the hands-on caregivers, who handle some of the most unpleasant but critical tasks such as helping with personal hygiene, changing adult briefs, or helping with mouth care. Professional caregivers can be subjected to very challenging behaviors, especially when residents have dementia. Plus, they may encounter difficult personalities, some of which can be rude and even mean. Many caregivers in these communities work long hours and are not paid well. Some even work two or three jobs. However, as the saying goes, one bad apple can spoil the whole bunch. And this is true for all professions. There may be some bad apples. However, if you can come to appreciate and value the staff in these communities and show them that you care about them, they will be happier and will be more likely to provide better care. And you will pave the way to becoming a more successful partner in care.

My Story

Becoming a partner in care whether your care recipient is in a nursing home or assisted living facility helps ensure better care for your care recipient. However, another extremely valuable aspect is that *you too* often benefit. Let me share my story and then summarize how being a partner in care can impact your own self-care.

My mother lived for many years in long-term care facilities and here's what I did to partner in care. First off, I did my best to get to know all my mother's primary caregivers, both nurses and nurse assistants. I shared as much information as I could that would help them best care for her.

Each time I visited, I would bring a picture of Mom during a certain time period in her life. I would share it with all the staff that day and then place it on the bulletin board in her room. I wanted them to really know my mother, not just who she was now but also who she had been. In addition, I believed it was important for me to get to know the staff as best as I could. I asked questions about them, where they were born, where they grew up, if they had a family, and what they enjoyed doing. I also learned that many caregivers worked two and three jobs. This by itself made me appreciate all they did and how hard they worked. I thought of different ways to show my gratitude. My mother loved pizza. So on her birthday, I would order pizza for each shift and take turns each year having a lunch or dinner-time pizza party. My mother also loved ice cream. So when I would bring my mother an ice cream sundae from the local fast food restaurant, I would bring sundaes for all her caregivers. Not only were the staff appreciative, I learned that several caregivers would go to the fast food restaurant and buy Mom a sundae with their own money.

Talk about being a partner in care! I was so touched. I immediately left an envelope with money in which the caregivers could use to buy Mom and themselves something when they went on a fast food run. All of these things helped my mother receive excellent compassionate care. And I felt less stressed and more at ease because I didn't have to worry about my mother. When I went on vacations, instead of feeling horribly guilty, the caregivers would immediately reassure me that they would take good care of my mom while I was away and not to worry! As you can see, there are many opportunities and benefits to being a partner in care, including:

- You can feel more confident that the staff knows your care recipient, which can provide you with a *sense of relief.*
- The staff members feel to you as if they are part of your "extended family." This can help lessen your worry and guilt—two major issues that many caregivers face.
- You may experience more joy because you feel more comfortable with the staff, and vice versa.
- You can feel more at ease because the staff members inform you of the positive situations with your care recipient, not just the negative ones. You come to realize that it truly does take a village to care for one another.

There are many advantages of being a partner in care, let's now examine how to be a positive advocate.

ADVOCATING MATTERS

> You can do all the right things, but if they're done for the wrong rea-
> sons or with the wrong attitude, your efforts will be short-circuited.
> —Mark Sandborn, *The Fred Factor*, 110

As was mentioned early in this chapter, advocacy goes hand in hand with partnering in care. Too often, however, caregivers think about advocacy as having to handle problems. Certainly there are times when this is the case. But I have seen how *not partnering* with the staff can set caregivers up for fear, worry, and frustration. This, in turn, can set you up to be more confrontational than you intended. The next section highlights some of the most common challenges that may require advocacy. Before I address those, however, I want to discuss ways to be a positive advocate for your care recipient. It requires a mindfulness approach in which you stay present through each challenge. It's easy to become overwhelmed with all that you have to do and the problems that inevitably arise. As a mindful advocate, you recognize the importance of staying as calm as you can. When you do so, you are less likely to be confrontational. You can approach staff members by what I call a "care-fronting" way. When you *care-front*, you advocate with the intention of being calm, clear, and present. Your goal is to work cooperatively with staff so you can obtain the best outcome for you and your care recipient. You learn how to prioritize your concerns and take on one challenge at a time. Utilizing a care-front approach is a skill that takes practice and patience. Yet the rewards from your effort will be exceedingly positive.

The next sections address how to advocate when your care recipient moves into a long-term care environment. I have created separate sections on being an advocate in assisted living facilities and nursing homes because there are some rather different tasks needed.

Advocating in Assisted Living Facilities

Your role as advocate in an assisted living facility is to be aware of the *most common problems* so you can be proactive and even prevent them from occurring. As you are aware, in any human service environment, problems and issues can occur. The following are some of the most common issues and my suggestions on what to be aware of and how to handle them.

Voicing Your Concerns

When you have repeatedly expressed your concerns and nothing appears to be changing, there are several different actions you can try as a positive advocate. For example, start with a discussion with the *nurse in charge of the day-to-day care*. She is generally most informed about your care recipient's health issues. However, if you have serious care concerns, then talk to the *nurse manager or supervisor*. If your care issues are still not being resolved, set up an appointment with the *executive director*. And if there still is no resolution that is comfortable to you, call the *regional director* for the assisted living company, if they have one. Most assisted living facilities are part of larger companies and therefore have managers at the regional or even national level. Lastly, you can always call the *ombudsman* of that community. An ombudsman is a consumer advocate who works for the state and is responsible for investigating and resolving complaints. Most assisted living communities have an ombudsman assigned to their facility. The ombudsman of the facility your care recipient is living in will attempt to work collaboratively with you and with the facility to help come up with a solution.

Medications

It is very important that the facility keeps track of medications, administers them properly, and informs you of any changes. I suggest you request a medication activities record (MAR) for your records. A MAR is the way the facility keeps track of the medications your care recipient is on. Request a copy of the MAR at least a couple of times a year or when your care recipient has been in the hospital. MARs are particularly pertinent if your care recipient has many prescriptions or had recent changes in medications. If your care recipient is getting a new medication, make sure you get an explanation of what the medication is, what it is for, and what to expect. If the prescription is for an emotional or behavioral issue, inquire about what staff members have done to try to alleviate the problem. Also, keep close track of the billing for these medications. I have seen clients charged for medications that the care recipient is no longer using.

Emotional and Behavioral Issues

What is the best way for the facility to handle emotional and/or behavioral issues with your care recipient? The answer to this question is tricky. Ideally, emotional and or behavioral issues can be lessened through the many benefits of a good assisted living community. First, there are a number of staff members who can interface with your care recipient and share the "care challenges," so to speak. And in the better facilities, caregivers are trained how to handle emotional and behavioral issues with residents. Another benefit of an assisted living community is the many opportunities for socialization, which can also help alleviate boredom, isolation, or depression. Find out if your care recipient is attending activities, and whenever possible, attend an activity with her.

Medication and Emotional or Behavioral Issues

There is no doubt that medication can and should be used for some people and for some situations. It is also important to be mindful that some facilities and clinicians overuse medications. If you are considering medications for emotional or behavioral issues, find out if the facility works with a geriatric physician or geriatric psychiatrist. If the facility doesn't have a consulting geriatric doctor, it will be prudent that you find a doctor experienced in prescribing for elders. Given properly, medication can be very helpful and can positively impact your care recipient's quality of life and help staff provide the best possible care.

Accusations

Sometimes your care recipient will tell you about things that aren't going well at his facility. By all means, check them out. But if your care recipient has dementia, then advocating is a little different. Be mindful that he has less cognitive awareness and can't always speak for himself or give you correct information. For example, he may tell you he hasn't had lunch when in fact he just did, or that someone is stealing his belongings. It's important to check out with staff members whether your care recipient's perspective is accurate.

ER Visits and Hospitalization

Make sure you understand what, if any, clinicians or nurses are available at your care recipient's assisted living facility and what their particular policies are with regards to dealing with illness, falls, or urgent health situations. Some of the potential reasons that your care recipient would need emergency care include a possible broken bone from a fall, sudden change in health status (e.g., low blood pressure), or significant discomfort or pain. When there is a health concern that may require an emergency room visit, the nurse should carefully assess your care recipient. If the facility does not have a registered or licensed practical nurse, ask about the procedure for assessing residents. Also, let them know your preferred hospital and make sure it is listed in your care recipient's chart.

Changes in Levels of Care

It's important to ask *up front*, and if possible before you admit your care recipient, how they determine changing the levels of care and how they inform you. A change in the level of care should ensue from increased needs for your care recipient. As explained in chapter 6, "Navigating the Maze of Professional Resources, Services, and Support," there can be many reasons for a change in care. Before a level of care change occurs, a clinical assessment should be conducted on your care recipient and the results shared with you verbally and in writing. If you disagree with the assessment, ask to have an outside consultant conduct an assessment. If you still dispute it, you may need to contact the ombudsman for the assisted living facility.

Memory Care

When your care recipient enters assisted living, it is possible that staff, at some point, may recommend that your care recipient be moved into the memory care part of the community. The biggest reason your care recipient would be moved is for safety. This includes engaging in any types of behaviors that put him at risk, such as wandering out of the facility. Other reasons for moving your care recipient are a need for additional assistance and supervision or because he is exhibiting unsuitable behaviors. An example of the latter includes nonsensical speech, taking clothes off, or eating meals with fingers. Your care recipient should be assessed appropriately and the results explained to you.

Caregivers definitely struggle with the notion of moving their care recipient into memory care. Caregivers worry that the other residents in memory care may be more impaired than their care recipient. And some may be. This can lead to worrying that your care recipient will decline even more quickly. Yet in most circumstances, this does not happen in reputable memory care programs. In fact, I have found that caregivers have a more difficult time adjusting to memory care than their care recipient does. Remember, be open to new opportunities and let go of how things used to be.

If the memory care program is properly supervised and provides meaningful activities, your care recipient can actually do better. Let me explain why. First, many assisted living residents are not always so kind to those who have cognitive problems. I have witnessed numerous examples of residents being outright mean and disparaging to a person with cognitive impairment. And being subjected to this type of treatment is demoralizing and can create additional stress. It is not unusual for a person to begin to isolate herself, realizing she can't keep up cognitively like she used to. She may also become depressed, anxious, and angry or agitated with you, other family members, or staff. Additionally, this becomes the time to really make sure you create a "circle of support" around your care recipient. The more she has loving, caring people around her, the better for you and her!

Evicting Residents

Caregivers often ask if their care recipient can be asked to move out of an assisted living facility. It's very important to carefully read the resident agreement, which should spell out the terms and conditions for discharge. In general, there are several reasons your care recipient may be asked to leave. The first is for nonpayment of fees. The second and more common reason is that your care recipient requires a higher level of care than the facility is licensed to provide. Your care recipient has a right to be given thirty days' notice, unless it is a health emergency or your care recipient is a danger to himself or others. If your care recipient requires a higher level of care than the facility is licensed to provide, the facility may apply for a waiver from the state. If granted, this would permit the facility to keep your care recipient. When this happens, I often see families paying for extra caregivers—sometimes as much as twenty-four/seven.

Well, now that you are armed with information for assisted living environments, let's move to advocating in nursing homes.

Advocating and Nursing Homes

Nursing home care presents a different kind of challenge for caregivers. The nursing home population is much frailer and often at the end stages of their diseases, which makes the care provided more complicated. As an advocate and partner, you are a crucial link in your care recipient's care. I hope the information below will help you feel more empowered and confident in advocating for the best care. As your care recipient's advocate, *be involved, don't accept the status quo, and don't be afraid to voice your concerns.* Here are several important considerations.

- *Stay connected to your care recipient.* You can learn a lot by participating in activities as well. For example, you can make sure that the activities are appropriate for your care recipient's abilities and also gauge whether your care recipient is participating in or enjoying them.
- *Visit on different days and times,* so you can get a sense of how the staff members on different shifts provide care. For instance, does the staff on all shifts appear to provide similar care? Are there changes in how many staff members are available? It isn't unusual to have fewer staff members at night.
- *Become a partner in care.* Caregivers generally have about eight to ten residents they are responsible for on their shift and most try to somehow provide person-centered care. (Person-centered care is care that is specific to your care recipient.) Give them the best information possible about your care recipient. And help them! Caregivers have told me how much they appreciate families who help them out on occasion. It might be escorting your care recipient to an activity or to the dining room. Or cutting up his food, if you visit during mealtime. I have found that when staff members view you as a true partner in care, they are even more willing to provide good care.

- *Get to know the various professionals in the system.* Try to meet all the department heads whenever possible. Ask questions. Ask how they communicate to you any problems or concerns. Find out who is the administrator on duty on the weekends in case of an emergency.
- *Participate in the care plan meetings.* Care plan meetings are fifteen- to twenty- minute meetings between the facility staff, you, other family members, and when appropriate, your care recipient. Staff from the facility usually includes a care plan coordinator, a social worker, dietary director, charge nurse, the activities director, and possibly other professionals who are involved in specialized care for your care recipient. The goal of the care plan meetings is to make sure that the best possible holistic care is being given to your care recipient. Each department responsible for providing services and care updates the goals that are mandated by the state after admission and then on a regular basis, usually quarterly. In addition, care plan meetings should be scheduled if your care recipient's medical condition has changed dramatically or he's been hospitalized. Care plan meetings provide you with the opportunity to ask questions, voice any concerns you may have, and hear how things are going with your care recipient. If you can't physically attend the meeting, ask to participate by telephone or request a different time to meet.
- *Know when to hospitalize.* As with assisted living facilities, it is important to understand the nursing home's procedures with regard to sending your care recipient to the ER or hospital. Likewise, it is important to let the facility know your preferences with regards to hospitalization. If you want your care recipient hospitalized, let them know which hospital. Alternatively, if you don't want your care recipient hospitalized, let them know you prefer that medical care be provided in the facility. The good news about nursing homes is that they are able to handle more challenging medical issues than assisted living facilities. Typically, nursing homes are staffed with a medical director and around-the-clock nursing staff, and can perform many diagnostic tests, such as blood tests, urinalysis, and x-rays.
- *Reinforce the good!* I can't stress enough the importance of complimenting staff members when they are providing kind, loving care. Too often, we all focus on the problems. Try to look for what *is* working. And when you see that, make sure you point it out.
- *Express your concerns.* I encourage you to express your concerns, as staff can't intervene if they aren't aware of what is troubling you. I know that this suggestion can evoke fear and trepidation in some caregivers. Many have shared that they are afraid to complain and worry that the care staff will take offense and take it out on their care recipient. Mindful caregivers recognize that it is not what you say but how you say it. You can be assertive without being aggres-

sive. Or as I mentioned earlier in this chapter, you learn how to "care-front." Be clear, factual, and try to maintain a calm presence by managing your emotions. Often, your emotions get in the way of being an effective advocate.

- *Pick your battles.* Although this was mentioned above, it is worth mentioning again. Learn to pick which battles are the most important. If staff members experience you as a "complainer" or someone who is "never happy," you can be labeled as a "problem" caregiver. This, in turn, can sometimes create less incentive for staff to provide good care. I am not saying you shouldn't complain, just choose your battles and be mindful how you present your concern.
- *Know your rights.* You have the right to voice grievances. It's important to find out how to best voice your grievances. The nursing home may have a protocol they have set forth. With that said, I highly encourage you to develop a relationship with the charge nurse on each shift and the caregivers primarily responsible for your care recipient's care. Those particular staff members are usually in contact with your care recipient every day.
- *Troubleshoot your concerns.* If you have followed the nursing home's protocols for grievances and still feel as if your concerns have not been resolved, then you may have to contact the ombudsman of the facility in order to achieve a resolution amenable to everyone. Write down your specific concerns, state them clearly and factually, provide dates and if possible times of day the problem seems to be taking place. Most likely a meeting will be set up with you, the ombudsman, and several key staff members. Be prepared to discuss what you would like to accomplish from the meeting. And keep in mind that there will be situations in which your expectations and theirs may be different. To be a partner in care requires mindfully listening to their side, offering solutions along with hearing theirs, and before the meeting is over, making sure there are clear expectations and follow-up actions.

Molly Moves Sylvia into a Nursing Home

Sylvia needed to be moved into a nursing home in order to get around-the-clock care. Molly was an active advocate and partner in care. At the most recent care plan meeting, it was noted that Sylvia was losing some weight and seemed weak. The dietician suggested that Sylvia be weighed weekly, instead of monthly. The dietician also recommended that Sylvia be given protein shakes. Molly made sure the staff were weighing her mother and asked that they include more of Sylvia's favorite foods as part of her meals. She suggested adding chocolate pudding, chocolate yogurt, and peanut butter crackers as snacks and dessert. Molly also asked whether her mother needed some physical therapy to build up her endurance and stamina. A PT evaluation was done and PT was started. With the extra food, Sylvia's weight stabilized. Molly realized the importance of her being a positive advocate throughout her mother's stay in the nursing home.

Possible Medical Challenges

Before leaving this section, I'd like to discuss some of the most common medical problems that I have seen in nursing homes. Below are descriptions of the problems, as well as issues and solutions that you should be mindful of. I hope my suggestions will be helpful.

Pressure Sores

Pressure sores, or bed sores as they are commonly called, are an area of damaged skin usually caused by staying in a position for too long. Movement and rotating your care recipient's body helps with circulation and is critical to helping prevent pressure sores. If pressure sores are present, they most frequently occur in the buttocks, on elbows, and heels. Your care recipient is at most risk if she is bedridden, or is in a wheelchair and unable to change her position. There are other medical issues that can cause skin breakdown and lead to pressure sores. Pressure sores can cause serious infections, some of which can be life threatening. As an advocate, you will have to stay on top of this issue, particularly in nursing homes.

Urinary Tract Infections (UTIs)

Urinary tract infections are more common in older adults, especially those who reside in nursing homes. There are a variety of reasons, including poor hygiene, improper hydration, and kidney problems. What is crucial for caregivers to understand is that UTIs can cause symptoms of dementia. I've seen UTIs cause confusion, disorientation, agitated behavior, and paranoia. And if your care recipient already has dementia, he may experience more profound confusion, agitation, or other behavioral symptoms. Your care recipient may also experience painful urination or pain in her lower abdomen and may not be able to express how she feels. You may notice she is having trouble sitting still or seems to grimace a fair amount. There can also be a strong urine odor. Be proactive and let the charge nurse know if you suspect something. Being aware of the symptoms of a UTI can potentially prevent them from getting worse or misdiagnosed. When UTIs are undetected, care recipients can be given inappropriate medications to treat the behavioral symptoms instead of the underlying problem and, even more critical, you can potentially prevent unnecessary hospitalizations. More often than not, when UTIs are not detected, the infection can become so severe that your care recipient would need to be hospitalized.

Hygiene

Hygiene is one of the biggest challenges caregivers face in nursing homes. Hygiene can involve elimination, mouth care, and bathing. If you encounter hygiene problems, it will be important for you to determine the cause. Sometimes the reasons are staff related, such as staff shortages, inadequate supervision, or even unwillingness. Sometimes the reasons are with the resident, who can refuse care or even become combative and aggressive.

It is common that when a person is admitted to a nursing home, she most likely will be incontinent of bladder and sometimes even bowel. Incontinence and hygiene issues often go hand in hand. If your care recipient is not changed or cleaned up appropriately, he can develop UTIs and skin breakdown, which can lead to pressure sores. Care recipients should not be left in soiled briefs. Caregivers should check your care recipient every couple of hours to make sure he is clean and dry. If this is not happening, address it immediately.

Another hygiene challenge is mouth care. If your care recipient's teeth and mouth are not attended to properly, he can develop all sorts of dental problems, including serious infections. You should be able to detect some problem if you notice your care recipient's breath seems bad. There are residents who absolutely will not let caregivers clean their teeth. They bite down on the toothbrush or are unwilling to open their mouth. There are ways to resolve this, including mouth rinses and alternative toothbrushes that are less invasive.

Lastly, there can be care recipients who will refuse to bathe. Telltale signs are body odor and unclean hair. There are ways to resolve this as well—try a shower instead of a bath or use a sponge bath. And think about ways you can be a partner in care. Talk with staff members and find out if there might be other ways to help. For example, you might be able to wash your care recipient's hair, or if not, perhaps no rinse soap would help.

Dehydration

Dehydration is a very common problem among nursing home residents. First off, care recipients may refuse to drink fluids or may have problems swallowing. Second, caregivers may not always make sure that their care recipient is drinking enough. I recommend the following. Ask that some sort of fluid or food high in water content be given to your care recipient every few hours. And also request that they make sure your care recipient is actually ingesting it. Too many times I have found food or drinks just sitting untouched in the resident's room. In addition, you might bring some foods or drinks that your care recipient really enjoys. For instance, I brought over different kinds of soups and fruits for my mother, which was a great way to get liquids into her. And whenever anyone else comes to visit, they should do the same.

Nutrition

A common fear I hear from families and caregivers is that their care recipient is not being fed enough or given sufficient time in which to eat. There are a couple of things to look for to determine if this is in fact the case. The most obvious is weight loss. Nursing homes residents are supposed to be weighed monthly. Ask to see his chart and his weight. If you are concerned, ask that he be weighed more frequently and request a meeting with the director of dietary. You can partner with her by possibly recommending some foods that could be added to your care recipient's diet. As was suggested above, eat with your care recipient as much as possible. And ask other visitors to bring food or also share a meal as well. I'd like to add one solemn note about nutrition. Be aware that when a person is close to the end stages of her disease, she may begin to take in less food. If this is the case, it will be important to discuss what actions are the most appropriate. This many also include hospice, which is discussed in the next chapter.

Bottom line, when you have a care recipient in a nursing home, you will most likely have to advocate at one time or another. Be as proactive as possible, and know the extent to which improvement or recovery is possible so you can have realistic expectations and become a partner in care.

ADVOCATING AND BEING A PARTNER IN CARE

"Why Can't My Husband Ever Look Good?"

Rachel's husband, Tom, had been in the nursing home for about two months, Tom had dementia. She had been caring for him in her home by herself for almost four years, but his dementia had progressed and he had become more difficult to care for. As she told me, "I succumbed to placing him in a nursing home." The day Rachel came to see me, she was completely distraught. Every time she visited Tom, she found him unshaven and his hair uncombed. Tom had been a meticulous dresser and had always been well groomed. Rachel said the situation was "killing her" and that she felt horribly guilty. She wondered if she should take Tom back home. I asked how she expressed her concerns to the staff. She said that after talking with the charge nurse about Tom's grooming, he would look better for a few days, but they couldn't seem to keep him that way. After talking with Rachel, I learned that she enjoyed certain aspects of caring for her husband and missed doing some of those things for him. We discussed how she could become a "partner in care" and positive advocate. With my encouragement, she asked for a meeting with the caregiver and charge nurse. She calmly explained the importance of her husband looking as "spiffy" as possible. She shared some of her care tips and asked if she could help with some of his care. Together, they decided that she could be in charge of Tom's haircuts and could shave him and style his hair when she visited him. Additionally, I encouraged Rachel to compliment the staff when her husband looked well groomed. Rachel made it a point to let the caregivers know how great he looked and how much it meant to her. Within a month, her husband's grooming improved. And the relationship with the caregivers improved as well. She became a true partner in care.

Sylvia's Next Transition

Sylvia had been in the nursing home for almost a year when her health took a turn for the worse. Her body just was giving out. Because Molly had become a great partner in care and advocate for Sylvia, she and the care staff decided together to bring in hospice care. The nursing home worked with several local hospice organizations and Molly interviewed them all and chose one to help her and her mother. For several months, Sylvia received additional medical support to control the pain and keep her comfortable. Molly took advantage of the hospice's spiritual and emotional counseling. Sylvia passed peacefully with Molly at her side.

I hope this chapter has inspired you to be mindful of the incredible benefits of being a partner in care and advocate for your care recipient. The next chapter offers information and ideas about how to help your care recipient "finish well."

NOTES

1. Zhanlian Feng, Brad Wright, and Vincent Mor, "Sharp Rise in Medicare Enrollees Being Held in Hospitals for Observation Raises Concerns about Causes and Consequences," *Health Affairs* 31, no. 6 (2012).

EIGHT

When the End Is Near

Finishing Well

> Grief arises because we are not alone and what connects us to others
> and to the world also breaks our hearts.
> —Miriam Greenspan, *Healing through the Dark Emotions*, 45

The death of a loved one is one of the most profound losses caregivers
can experience, and sooner or later, they will realize there is no way to
escape this loss. Death can throw us off balance. It affects us emotionally,
physically, spiritually, and socially. Losing, being left, and having to let
go are all a part of the caregiving journey. Some caregivers will experience these losses as life altering, adding new meaning and value to their
lives. Other caregivers may experience these losses as devastating, bringing with them overwhelming sadness and suffering. Although loss and
grief are constant companions, caregivers will find they can be humbled
by both. The experience, however, can provide opportunities to embrace
faith, blessings, and love.

This chapter offers insight and understanding so that when you come
face to face with loss, and ultimately death, you will be better able to
cope. You will learn ways to approach loss so you have the opportunity
to "finish well." Finishing well is a concept coined by family therapist Dr.
Terry Hargrave.[1] Finishing well requires being conscious of your losses
and how they affect you. To finish well, you must work on your unfinished business. The most common barrier to finishing well is unfinished
business. For caregivers, unfinished business is when you have regrets,
harbored anger, or resentment toward your caregiving situation. Unfinished business can wreak havoc on your mind, body, and spirit. It interferes with being able to process your grief. While you may not be able to
revolve all your unfinished business, the critical issue is being able to find

163

ways to make peace with it. When you are able to reconcile your unfinished business, you have a much greater opportunity to "finish well."

UNDERSTANDING LOSS AND GRIEF

People die, but love does not die. It is recycled from one heart, from one life, to another.
                           —Harold Kushner, *Living a Life That Matters,* 125

It takes great courage to acknowledge loss and grief. We live in a culture that emphasizes feeling good and tends to push aside feelings that are painful or unhappy. Thus many people are uncomfortable talking about death. Yet, we all know that living life means living loss. The following section explains the different losses you may experience and how you can become stuck in the grieving process. Becoming more familiar with these issues can help you proceed down a path of a healthier grieving.

As you read these various sections, be aware that each of us has to find our own unique way of grieving. This requires finding ways to find some time for mindfulness exploration. Focus on yourself and the array of feelings that come forth as you process your grief and loss. You may find that reflection, meditation, and prayer are ways to explore your feelings. Or you may feel more comfortable writing some of your feelings down. When you take the time to process your feelings, you will be more likely to journey through this stage of caregiving with more ease.

DEFINITION OF LOSS, GRIEF, MOURNING, AND BEREAVEMENT

Let's examine the terms associated with the grieving process and how they can affect you. *Loss* is the reaction to losing something that has meaning and value to you. Even though losses can be great or small, they all require that you acknowledge and process your feelings about them. *Grief* is the reaction to the loss and involves a wide range of feelings and emotions. Each caregiver will experience grief in his own unique way. Some of you will be more private and quiet with your grief, and others will need to express grief to friends, family, and perhaps even to professionals. *Bereavement* refers to the period of intense emotions and feelings you have after you experience the loss. The bereavement period can be the most uncomfortable time for you, as you are immersed in your grief and generally feel your pain more acutely. You also may feel more disorganized and out of sorts. While this period of time is difficult, it usually lasts only a month or two. *Mourning* is the way you process your grief and loss. Mourning can last several months or even several years. The bereavement and mourning process is important because it provides the space to heal the loss. Mindful caregivers make room for grief and recognize the importance of honoring it.

DIFFERENT WAYS YOU CAN EXPERIENCE LOSS

For caregivers, there are several different ways you may experience loss and grief. Understanding this process helps to normalize your feelings and can help you cope in healthier ways.

- *Sudden Loss*: This type of loss occurs out of the blue, is unexpected, can't be anticipated, and happens immediately or very quickly. The response to this loss is often shock, disbelief, denial, and overwhelming feelings. An example might be that your care recipient dies suddenly from a stroke or heart attack. Caregivers who experience sudden loss can feel as if they were hit by a Mack truck. Coping with sudden loss is generally very difficult, because there is no opportunity for closure. Closure allows a chance to say goodbye and express your feelings with the person before she dies. Without the opportunity to express your feelings, you may feel cheated, robbed, and angry. Thus, with sudden loss you may have a much more difficult time processing your grief.
- *Uncertain Loss*: In this situation, the loss is unclear because you do not know if the person is going to live or die. An example would be when a care recipient has had a stroke or is in a coma. You don't know how long your care recipient will remain in this uncertain condition. Coping with uncertain loss creates a great deal of ambiguity and can bring forth all kinds of mixed emotions. Uncertain loss can create a great deal of stress for caregivers and interfere with relationships outside the caregiving situation. When caregivers have to cope with this type of loss, it can feel like an endless journey. Some caregivers report feeling angry and frustrated; others feel helpless and hopeless. Still others express overwhelming sadness or anxiety. Many caregivers say they feel as if they are on a constant roller-coaster. Unfortunately, managing your emotions and finding ways to cope with uncertain loss is not easy.
- *Certain Loss*: This involves a situation in which loss is inevitable and predictable, usually from a terminal and incurable illness. Chronic disease, certain cancers, Alzheimer's disease, Parkinson's, and certain serious injuries all fall into this category. With this type of loss, it is important to be aware that caregivers have time for closure. You have a chance to process your grief and attempt to work through some of your unfinished business. Certain loss provides the opportunity to process your grief.

Normal Grieving

> And ever has it been that love knows not its own depth until the hour
> of separation.
>   —Kahil Gibran, *The Collected Works*, 99

In the caregiving world, there is no way to escape loss. As one caregiver shared with me, "My job as caregiver is to learn to navigate through the great sea of loss. As one wave hits me and I regain my balance and recover, I get hit with another." There are certainly times when many of you may feel the same way. Understanding what are normal and abnormal ways of grieving can help caregivers ride these waves with more ease.

First, let's explore what is meant by *normal grieving*. Normal grieving involves acknowledging the loss so you can process your feelings and move forward. When you allow yourself to grieve, you are better able to process your feelings and cope more effectively. Dr. Elisabeth Kûbler-Ross, an authority on death and dying, identified five different states that people experience going through the dying process.[2] Subsequent years of research have resulted in other experts adding new insights. I have also added my own and explained how these states can affect caregivers. Being mindful of these common sets of issues can help validate your feelings and potentially alleviate some stress and discomfort. Increased understanding and knowledge can often make you feel more empowered.

Shock and Denial

You find out that your care recipient has been diagnosed with a chronic disease, disability, or terminal illness. The diagnosis can bring forth feelings of shock and denial because the information often comes as a surprise, is overwhelming, and is hard to digest. Usually within a week or two, you are able to assimilate the information and acknowledge the impending loss.

Bargaining

Many of us will come up with some sort of deal or agreement that we hope will change the inevitable outcome. While you can acknowledge the loss, at the same time, you feel the need to hold onto hope. You may consider praying to God or a higher power, asking for the possibility that your care recipient could get better. Or you might ask for forgiveness, particularly if you feel that you could have been more compassionate or patient toward your care recipient.

Anger

When the denial wears off, it can sometimes be replaced by fury and rage at the situation. These feelings sometimes surprise caregivers. You may notice that you become very impatient with your care recipient and with yourself and others. And when you internalize your anger, you can become either depressed or anxious, or both.

Depression

Depression is a common state for many caregivers. This stage is characterized by feeling incredibly sad, out of control, and depressed. You now are getting more in touch with what you expect to lose and how your life will change. For some caregivers, depression becomes even more pronounced because they have isolated themselves from those they love. In this stage, you may feel even more depleted, both physically and emotionally. You also may find it difficult to concentrate and care for your care recipient.

Acceptance

Acceptance means you are able to recognize the loss and accept its finality. You have to find ways to grieve and let go, so that you can eventually create a new life without your care recipient. In my practice, I have noticed that many caregivers struggle emotionally with this stage.

Accommodation

I talk with caregivers about the idea of *accommodating* their loss instead of acceptance. I like the word "accommodate" because it infers that a process will take place and that this process can take some time. Accommodating the loss allows you to slowly move toward acceptance. It recognizes that your grief may resurface at times, even many years after your care recipient has died. Accommodating also helps you concede that you may not be able to quite get to acceptance.

Anticipatory Grieving

> "It seems that just when I get used to one loss, I have to cope with the next. The hardest part about being with my mother through Alzheimer's disease is losing my mother in little bits."
>
> —A daughter

Many caregivers who read this quote are probably able to identify with this daughter. Caring for someone with a chronic disease means you most likely will be caring for them for many years. In most circumstances, you will experience loss each time your care recipient declines. Anticipatory grieving is the process by which you begin to let go and say goodbye in small bites while your care recipient is still alive. *Anticipatory grieving* is a normal part of grieving. For example, when caring for someone who has Alzheimer's disease, you may experience continual loss — labeled by many caregivers as "the long goodbye." As your care recipient loses more abilities, you have to adjust to more losses, which seem to endure throughout the illness. It can really feel like a "long goodbye"! These losses make you more aware that your relationship and roles with your care recipient will continually change. It takes courage to acknowledge these changes and even greater courage to adjust to them. Being a mindful caregiver encourages you to embrace the anticipatory grieving process. When you give yourself the space to experience your grief along the way, you can cope in more positive ways.

Abnormal Grieving

> Grief is a wound that needs attention in order to heal.
> —Judy Tatelbaum, *The Courage to Grieve*, 9

In contrast to the many normal states people experience, let's now talk about *abnormal grieving*. It should come as no surprise that many caregivers will be challenged by abnormal grieving, or what I sometimes call unhealthy grieving Unhealthy grieving is experiencing grief but not acknowledging or processing it. This can result from a variety of reasons and circumstances, including denial about the impending loss of your care recipient, burying yourself in your caregiving duties, not tending to self-care, or not making time to process the grief.

Ask yourself if any of the following situations describe you. If so, they can set you up to experience abnormal grieving.

- Your *relationship* with your care recipient can impact how you will process grief. The following can make it much more difficult to process grief:

  1. You may have some unfinished business or emotional issues that have not been addressed.
  2. You may have a long history of not being close to your care recipient.
  3. Your care recipient may have been abusive.

- You may have been "cut-off," which is a family therapy term defined as intentionally not communicating with your care recipient. Now because your care recipient needs care, you are faced with being involved in her life.
- Your *care recipient's* medical condition, including:

  1. Your care recipient is in denial.
  2. Your care recipient has dementia.
  3. Your care recipient is extremely depressed.

- Your *own discomfort* with loss and death

    1. Perhaps you learned in your family that you just "get over" loss or death.
    2. You may be afraid of death, especially your own dying.

- You are so busy with life and caregiving

    1. Perhaps your own life situation, family, or job on top of caregiving gives you no time for yourself.

There are many different ways abnormal grief can rear its head, including delayed grief, complicated grief, and idealized grief. By describing these common states, my hope is that you will understand them and realize that there are healthy ways to work through them.

Delayed Grief

Delayed grief occurs when you don't allow yourself to fully process your loss. As a result, it can be years after your care recipient has died that your grief surfaces. Caregiving, in a sense, is the "perfect storm" for delayed grief. Some of you are so used to keeping busy and doing for your care recipient that you don't take time to acknowledge the various losses that are taking place. You either push aside your feelings or label them as unworthy of your attention. There are many ways delayed grief can impact caregivers, including depression and anxiety. Or, you may unintentionally take out some of your unexpressed feelings on others. The following is an example of a caregiver who experienced delayed grief and how she learned to work through it.

"I *Had* to Take Over the Business" — Spouse Caregiver, Frances

Dr. Murphy was caring for an elder woman who had panic attacks. After a complete physical to make sure there weren't any underlying medical issues, he prescribed anxiety medication and referred her to me. During our first session together, I learned that Frances's husband had died three years earlier. It wasn't until after her husband died that she began having panic attacks. When I asked how she coped with her husband's death, Frances answered, rather unemotionally, that she partook in the typical Jewish funeral rituals and then "had" to take over the family business. Frances also shared, however, that it was very hard for her to go to work. She felt terribly sad, yet she kept working because "that's what her husband would have wanted and expected."

It was clear that Frances's panic attacks were probably a result of not allowing herself to fully grieve over her husband's death. I explained delayed grief. By going right back to work, I told Frances, she didn't allow herself the time she needed to grieve. Frances looked dumbfounded and then started crying. She shared that the only time she had allowed herself to cry was at his funeral. Once Frances stopped crying, I suggested that it might be helpful to create some space to continue to process her grief. I asked if she could find some ways to honor her husband's memory and spirit. We discussed several different options, and she decided to pick out her favorite picture of her husband. So every morning and night, Frances would look at the picture and tell her husband how much she loved and missed him. When Frances came back a week later, she told me how much better she felt. Not one panic attack, although she admitted to a lot of tears. I reinforced that the tears would most likely lessen over time. Frances said that it felt good to talk to him, although she feared that people would think she was crazy talking to a picture. I told her it could be "our little secret," and she smiled.

As a caregiver, you need to be mindful that grieving takes time and requires acknowledgment of your feelings about your care recipient and to honor whatever relationship you have had. Each caregiver will have to determine what feels most comfortable. For some, it might be talking to your care recipient's picture, like Frances did. Others may need to light a candle in his memory or go to the cemetery. At the end of this chapter, I offer some additional rituals of remembering.

Complicated Grief

Complicated grief is grief that continues on well after the person has died. Often there is unfinished business that complicates the grief process. Complicated grief situations can greatly interfere with people's lives. Caregivers can feel totally overwhelmed by the loss, so much so that they can barely function. Those who have complicated grief struggle with just getting through their day-to-day lives. The following is an example of how an elder caregiver experienced complicated grief and how he coped.

"Why Didn't God Take Me?"—Mary Ann's Wish

Mary Ann came to me because her husband, Joe, was concerned that she was still struggling with the loss of her adult grandson, Billy, who had Down's syndrome. One of the first things Mary Ann said to me was, "Why didn't God take me instead?" Ever since their own daughter had died from cancer five years ago, Mary Ann and Joe had been caring for Billy. Since Billy's death a year earlier, Mary Ann had lost over twenty pounds and was continually sad. Mary Ann felt it had been her responsibility to do everything she could to make sure that Billy lived as long as he could. She had promised her daughter that no matter what, she would take care of him. Unfortunately, Billy contracted pneumonia and ended up dying. He was fifty years old.

In our session, the first thing Mary Ann said to me was, "I wished God would have taken me." No one could seem to comfort her. Mary Ann had some unfinished business over the death of her daughter, which was complicating the grieving related to her grandson. While Mary Ann was extremely sad about her daughter's death, she also harbored hidden anger about being responsible for her grandson. Once Mary Ann acknowledged and processed the leftover feelings, she was able to tackle the additional feelings about the death of her grandson. Mary Ann shared that she felt some relief when Billy died, because she worried that her grandson would outlive her and Joe. Yet at the same time, she felt guilty about having those feelings. It took several months to help Mary Ann work through all her grief, but she hung in there. In our last session, she was able to share her feelings with Joe. When Joe heard what she had been harboring, he turned and said, "Mary Ann, I thank God that he didn't take you."

As you can see, complicated grief has within it layers of unfinished business laced with unresolved feelings. Many who experience complicated grief also latch onto unrealistic expectations. Here are a few ways to release some of the feelings in order to help you process your grief in healthier ways. Open your heart to prayer and ask for trust and unconditional acceptance. Perhaps write down your feelings, maybe even as a short poem. Each of you will have to determine what is most comforting. And remember, you can reach out to professionals for support.

Idealized Grief

Idealized grief occurs when you hide your true feelings about your care recipient. You act as if everything between you and your care recipient is fine, and after your care recipient dies, you "pretend" that you are experiencing grief. Our culture expects that when you lose someone, you should feel sad and awful. Yet this may not be true for all caregivers. Some of you may have been caring for someone who was distant or even abusive. In these situations, you truly may not feel sad. Deep in your heart, you may even be relieved that your care recipient is gone. But because those feelings are not sanctioned by our culture, you may try to reframe your relationship in an "idealized" way. In other words, you try to convince yourself and others that your care recipient was wonderful and you will really miss him. Processing grief this way only serves to prolong your grief process and can cause you to become depressed, angry, or anxious. Here's an example of a spouse who struggled with idealized grief.

"Everyone Loved My Husband"—A Spouse's Struggle

Mable came to me by way of her daughter's encouragement. Mable's husband had been the minister of their church and was quite popular. He had died about a year earlier, and since then, Mable hadn't wanted to be around people, even her own family. Her daughter described her as nothing but depressed and short-tempered.

When Mable came into my office, she looked tired and unhappy. I asked her how she felt, and she said, "Oh, I am fine, but my daughter thinks I'm depressed." She quickly went on, "You know, everyone loved my husband, and people at church tell me all the time how much they miss him." Turning toward her, I said, "Well, do you miss him?" She quickly retorted, "Of course" and went on to say how fortunate she was to have married him. I wasn't so convinced. As Mable was sharing her story, something seemed amiss. I had a hunch that how everyone else felt about Mable's husband was not how Mable felt. After three sessions, Mable finally admitted that she had felt unappreciated by her husband. All her life, she had to listen to people telling her how wonderful her husband was. Yet what people didn't know was that he was mean, continually put her down, and told her that she was stupid and fat. The most difficult time of all, she said, was when he became ill and she had to take care of him.

No wonder Mable had to idealize her grief. I encouraged her to be mindful of her feelings, which were a mixture of relief, sadness, and guilt. I then worked with Mable to validate and normalize them. Once Mable was able to separate her own feelings from those of others, she realized she didn't need to idealize her husband any more. Her true feelings emerged, and she was able to process the sadness she felt for the relationship she wished she had but didn't. I wonder how many other caregivers may have had similar experiences.

Idealized grief is one of the trickiest situations to cope with. What's vital is that caregivers validate their feelings and give themselves permission to go against societal beliefs and pressures. An example would be admitting that after fifty years of marriage, you are relieved that your spouse has died. Another example might be acknowledging your resentment for having to care for your sister whom you were really not close to. In other words, you have to be willing to honor all of you, your dark and light sides. You have to let go of believing you have to feel a certain way. Once you honor who you are and stay congruent to yourself, you may find you don't have to idealize your grief.

DEMENTIA AND HOW IT COMPLICATES LOSS AND GRIEF

"Living with someone with dementia is akin to the long goodbye. Many times throughout my caregiving journey, I would say goodbye to another way I knew my husband."

—A spouse

Coping with AD or other forms of dementia has been described by many caregivers as "the long goodbye" or "the funeral that never ends." One of the great challenges of caring for someone with dementia is the continual loss and grief throughout the caregiving journey. This creates challenges that are different from those associated with other illnesses. The biggest difference is that you experience *ambiguous loss* (refer to chapter 3). Ambiguous loss is the uncertainty of what to expect each day from your care recipient's situation. For example, you are on a constant roller-coaster, never knowing how your care recipient's cognitive functioning will be moment to moment, day to day. Will he remember you today and allow you to help take care of him? Or will you be someone else he doesn't like? Will she resist your care and even your presence? Will he be agitated when you visit or will he be almost nonresponsive? Will she accuse you of trying to kill her with the medication you are giving her, or will she just take it with ease?

Living with these kinds of uncertainties can cause considerable anxiety, stress, and feelings of being out of control. Another way caregivers describe this ambiguity is feeling as if they experience "little deaths" that are hard to grieve. In fact, it can be very difficult for caregivers to acknowledge and express their grief about these losses when their care recipient is still alive. Thus, the challenges posed by ambiguous loss can cause additional wear and tear on caregivers emotionally, physically, and spiritually. Over the years, many caregivers in my practice have shared how they secretly wished their care recipient would "just die."

Caring for someone with dementia can feel like an "overdue death." An overdue death is labeled as a situation in which the person who has the chronic illness lives on even though his mind or body is barely functioning. Yet admitting these feelings to family or close friends can leave you feeling guilty and embarrassed. This leads to another major difference in coping with loss when caring for someone with dementia, the lack of societal understanding of what it is like living with this disease. This is called disenfranchised grief.

Disenfranchised Grief

Caring for someone with dementia can cause what professionals label as *disenfranchised grief*. Disenfranchised grief is the experience of feeling grief that is not recognized, understood, or legitimized by our culture. For example, a friend says, "Why do you go visit your mother, she doesn't recognize you anymore?" This kind of statement epitomizes *disenfranchised grief*. The situation is heartbreaking. Your mother's health is declining, and she doesn't remember you. You want to stay connected but know she's likely to die soon. Your friends may be confused by your grief. Dementia is ongoing and continually brings up uncomfortable feelings for a lot of people. The complexity it brings to relationships and how it impacts your life is not fully appreciated by the general culture. Caregivers may find that their friends do not know what to say or how to offer support. Some caregivers have even said that they feel abandoned by the medical professionals who tend to their care recipients.

Because the situation is difficult for most people to understand, caregivers can greatly benefit from talking to others. Dementia support groups can be wonderful places for caregivers to share feelings with others who are going through similar experiences. The other participants "get" what you are going through. They understand ambiguous loss and how crazy-making dementia can make you feel. For some of you, support groups can offer comfort and a place to safely grieve. For others, you may prefer the privacy of a counselor who can offer similar comfort and safety.

Traumatic Grief

Many professionals who work in the aging field recognize that dementia not only causes difficulty in processing grief but can also cause stress that lingers long after your care recipient has died. Professionals label this type of stress as *traumatic stress* reactions. A traumatic stress reaction is when you continue to conceal unresolved emotions after your care recipient has died. For example, on the one hand, you may feel relief that your care recipient has died, but, on the other hand, you experience overwhelming anxiety. The anxiety can be a result from the years of trauma from coping and caring for someone with dementia.

I share the above descriptions to help you better understand why you may feel the way you do. If these experiences sound familiar, it may be helpful to seek the help of a professional. Caring for someone with dementia is difficult. And for many caregivers, there is relief when their care recipient dies.

END-OF-LIFE CHOICES

We live in a society that values staying in control. Coping with loss and grief can only be accomplished by surrendering control, so we can make room to honor our emotions. As many caregivers would concede, however, this is easier said than done.

You have no control over how or when your care recipient will ultimately die. Yet you can control how you cope with end-of-life care and the choices involved. This section begins by exploring some of the fears that can interfere with making end-of-life choices. Once aware of your fears, you can more mindfully navigate through the various decisions needed.

So what might you be fearful of? The following are the most common caregiver fears:

- You may be afraid of your own feelings. The *what ifs* begin to emerge such as:

  1. What if you start crying and can't stop?
  2. What if you cry in front of your care recipient?
  3. What if you don't cry after your care recipient dies?
  4. What if you become so depressed you can hardly function?
  5. What if you haven't resolved some of your leftover feelings, which could include anger, resentment, or guilt?
  6. What if you can't find a way to forgive your care recipient?

- You may be afraid of death itself.

  1. Are you afraid of how your care recipient will die?
  2. Are you afraid to be with your care recipient when he dies?
  3. Are you afraid you won't be there when he dies?

- You may be afraid of letting go of your care recipient.

  1. Do you believe that if you let go, you—in a sense—are giving up hope?

- You may be afraid to admit that your care recipient is really ill and is close to death.

  1. Do you believe that if you consider hospice care it means that your care recipient is going to die?

- You may be afraid that if your care recipient is in a nursing home or assisted living community the staff will not provide compassionate end-of-life care.

These questions are very normal. But let's now add how to apply mindfulness to your situation. So often caregivers get stuck in fear because they don't take the time to pause and step back. Using mindfulness, you need to pause, step back, and just be with your feelings. After you create space to address your fears and you still feel overwhelmed, I would encourage you to find someone to help. This could be a counselor, chaplain, or even a support group. Traveling through this stage of your journey is not easy and it is not unusual that caregivers may need some additional support. Let's now look at what you need to know to tackle end-of-life issues.

Advanced Directives

End-of-life decisions will go more smoothly if you have the legal documents needed in order to honor your care recipient's desires at end of life. *Advanced directives* are documents that your care recipient signs giving one or two people the "power" to make decisions on his behalf when he is no longer able to do so. Each state is different, so it is important to know the laws regarding advanced directives for your particular residence. Make sure your legal document is "durable," which means that the document is valid when your care recipient has cognitive impairment. However, most advanced directives include the following:

- *Durable Power of Attorney for Finances* (POAF): A document that gives a caregiver the power to transact business on behalf of the care recipient when he is either physically or cognitively incapacitated.
- *Durable Power of Attorney for Health Care* (POAHC): A document that specifies what medical procedures your care recipient would like done if he becomes either physically or cognitively incapacitated. This includes being able to place him in a nursing home, assisted living community, or an inpatient hospice.
- *Living Will*: A document that indicates that when your care recipient is in a terminal condition he either desires no extraordinary means to save his life or desires that everything be done to save his life.
- *Do Not Resuscitate* (DNR): A document that states that your care recipient doesn't want to be resuscitated if his heart stops beating or if he stops breathing.
- *Do Not Intubate* (DNI): A document that states that your care recipient doesn't want to be placed on a ventilator.
- *Do Not Hospitalize* (DNH): A document that states your care recipient won't be taken to the hospital.

The DNR, DNI, and DNH all tend to be included as part of the health care POA document.

Advanced directives need to be in place *before* your care recipient becomes incapacitated.

I often get asked about how to get an elder parent to sign the advanced directives when he or she won't even talk about end-of-life care. This question is one of the most commonly asked questions and one that causes caregivers incredible angst. I wish there were a simple answer that would fit every situation, but there is not. Let me recap some potential resolutions offered in previous chapters. You may want to consider how the generational challenges can get in your way. While the Traditionalist generation tends to be very private about personal matters, they do tend to listen to professionals, especially doctors or clergy. If there is a way to enlist professional support, do so. Plus, sometimes a good friend, adult grandchild, or other family member can be more successful than you. Next, many elders don't really understand how the POA works or when it goes into effect. Try reassuring your care recipient that the POA only goes into effect when she isn't capable of making a decision. This can help them be more receptive to signing the documents. Lastly, make the point that if your care recipient won't give *you* POA, she might end up having a stranger making health care and financial decisions for her.

The following are common questions caregivers tend to ask about advanced directives:

Q: Who should draw up the POA documents?

A: In most cases, documents drawn up by lawyers are likely to serve you the best as attorneys should be familiar with their state laws and compose the documents accordingly. I tend to recommend elder law attorneys because they are generally more aware of and experienced in issues related to long-term care, power of attorney, and other end-of-life issues.

Q: What if I can't afford an attorney, what do I do?

A: If you cannot afford an attorney, contact your state or local Legal Aid office. Generally speaking, Legal Aid provides sliding scale services. However, your care recipient would have to qualify for those services.

Q: Can I use online legal documents?

A: With today's Internet age, many legal documents are available online. However, carefully check out the source and make sure they qualify as official documents in your particular state.

Q: Should we choose one or two people to serve as my father's POA for health care?

A: I strongly suggest one person serve as the POA for health care. If the care recipient wants two people, such as his two children, then I recommend one be primary and the other be secondary. The secondary person serves as POA in the event that the primary child is unwilling or unable to perform the assigned tasks.

Q: What happens when two people are designated as the health care POA and they don't agree?

A: When two people serve as the health care POA and they disagree with each other, their options are limited. If they cannot resolve their differences, they will need to go to court.

Q: What happens if the POA doesn't agree with the wishes set forth by the care recipient?

A: Legally, the POA must adhere to the directives set forth by the care recipient. The only way to go against a person's wishes would be to petition the court.

Q: What makes a good POA for health care?

A: I suggest that the health care POA be someone very familiar with the care recipient and her health and desires. Plus, I generally suggest that the POA be someone who lives close by. This is particularly important if your care recipient has cognitive impairment or is so ill that she can't advocate for herself.

Q: What do you do if your care recipient doesn't have a POA for finances or for health care and is either cognitively, psychologically, or physically incapacitated?

A: Unfortunately, in most cases if you don't have a POA for finances and health care, you will have to turn to the legal system and that usually requires guardianship. (Please refer to chapter 1 for detailed information about guardianship.) Sadly, I get this question a lot in my practice. A lawyer will be needed to help you navigate through this situation.

As you can see, having advanced directives in place can offer some ease in the caregiving journey. Let's now look at another important end-of-life care issue—hospice and palliative care.

Palliative and Hospice Care

Unfortunately, there is a lot of discomfort and misinformation about palliative and hospice care. Caregivers often don't feel comfortable discussing the subject, but it can make a huge difference in the quality of the life for the caregiver and the care recipient. I often begin this conversation by acknowledging the discomfort and the fear of giving up hope. I share the following information to help you make more informed decisions about when and how to use hospice or palliative care. First off, let's define each of these terms.

Palliative Care

Palliative care refers to the medical, emotional, and spiritual care and services designed to enhance comfort and improve the quality of life during the last phase of a person's life. The goal of palliative care is to anticipate, prevent, and relieve suffering so that your care recipient will be more comfortable. It is most often considered when your care recipient is in the later stages of his illness. Palliative care can be provided in many different settings, including at home, in an assisted living facility, and in a nursing home. In addition, many hospitals offer palliative care services.

You can request that your care recipient be considered for palliative care. I have found that not all doctors are familiar with palliative care and its many benefits. If you are going to consider palliative care, make sure the services are covered by your care recipient's medical or long-term care insurance, and you have a doctor's order if needed. Palliative care professionals can help design a care plan for your care recipient. In most situations, you and your care recipient will be assigned a team of professionals who can answer any questions you might have and help support you both emotionally and spiritually. The team is usually comprised of a nurse, social worker, chaplain, and physician. The care plan team closely supervises your care recipient, monitors his symptoms, and informs you about how the illness is progressing. They keep a close eye on your care recipient and can help you determine when hospice care would be appropriate. For many, palliative care will segue into hospice care as the illness progresses.

Hospice Care

Hospice is not a "death sentence" but more of a "life-affirming sentence" that honors the sanctity of life and helps people finish well. Before I define hospice care, I want to share many myths and ask if you believe any of these as well.

- Only your care recipient's doctor can recommend hospice care.
- Hospice care is only for those who have cancer.
- You must have only six months or less to live to qualify.
- You can only receive hospice care in your home.
- Hospice is not covered under insurance; you have to pay out of pocket.
- Hospice care = death.
- Placing your care recipient on hospice care is a death sentence.

Do you believe any of these statements? Let me discuss what hospice care is and is not and how it might help you with your situation. Hospice refers to both the philosophy and the specific services provided to those facing a terminal illness or condition. The goal of hospice is to manage symptoms, improve quality of life, and provide comfort and support to the care recipient and his family. Hospice is similar to palliative care in that there is usually a team of health professionals who provide care. This team is specially trained in working with death and dying. The one difference between palliative care and hospice it that hospice is typically used when medical treatment is no longer desired or cannot offer a cure. Hospice can be provided either in home, facility, or an inpatient hospice facility.

The services provided by hospice can be a lifeline for caregivers. Here are some the benefits you may find:

- *Information*: The hospice team can answer your medical questions and help inform you about where your care recipient is in the dying process.
- *Comfort*: Knowing that there is a team that specializes in providing care to someone who is dying can be extremely comforting. In addition, a major goal of hospice is to make sure your care recipient is comfortable. As a result, she is carefully monitored and pain control is of utmost importance.

- *Support*: Hospice provides a team of professionals who can support you, which can greatly lessen caregiver stress and anxiety at the end of life.
- *Spiritual Help*: You have the opportunity to talk with the hospice chaplain. There are just times when you need to talk with someone outside your close circle of friends and family. Hospice provides a safe place for you to explore your feelings.

Hospice Guidelines

Hospice is available to people who are in the end stages of their Parkinson's, Alzheimer's, and other chronic diseases. They all can potentially qualify for hospice care. However, there are very specific criteria guidelines used by most hospices. Generally speaking, hospice care is appropriate for people who are in the end stages of their diseases and who *appear* to have six months or less to live. Most hospices require that your care recipient meet certain criteria, including:

- Uncontrolled or extreme pain
- Respiratory distress
- Frequent dehydration
- Uncontrolled nausea and vomiting
- Intractable diarrhea
- Progressive weakness
- Significant weight loss within a certain period of time
- Frequent infections that require an ER visit or hospital stay
- Significant agitation or anxiety, which cannot only distress your care recipient but also make it difficult to provide care

Be aware that the criteria will vary some from hospice to hospice. Some of my clients have been turned down by one hospice only to be accepted by another. Thus it can be a bit confusing. I highly encourage caregivers to ask the hospice intake worker or admissions nurse what specific criteria they require in order for your care recipient to qualify.

Additionally, there are different guidelines for inpatient hospice care. Again, I encourage you to ask the hospice what specific criteria they use for their inpatient program. Most inpatient hospices require that your care recipient be in the end stages of her disease but also be very *unstable* and unable to be kept comfortable at her current residence. Often an inpatient hospice is able to stabilize your care recipient and help make her more comfortable because they have staff around the clock who are trained in comfort measures.

It is key that caregivers know that they don't have to "wait" for a doctor to recommend hospice care. Unfortunately, there are still a few doctors who are either uncomfortable with recommending hospice, just don't think about it, or want to do all they can to continue treating a

person. *You can ask* for a hospice evaluation. This is particularly important when your care recipient is in the hospital. It's been my experience
that some doctors order more treatment or rehabilitative care when it
might not be in the best interests of your care recipient's quality of life.
Later in this section, I provide an example of this situation. Hospice is
covered under Medicare, Medicaid, and most health insurance plans.
Some long-term care insurance plans will provide hospice benefits as
well. If you don't have health insurance, ask around as there are some
hospices that accept people with no insurance and limited income. I have
one last and important note about hospice care. It's important to do your
homework ahead of time. Research your options *before* your care recipient needs this kind of care. Find out what the different hospice services
offer, learn how they work, and understand their particular guidelines.

The following are a few examples of how hospice can be a supportive
and rich experience.

"I Graduated from Hospice" — Madeline

I met Madeline when she was ninety-two years young. Madeline had
always been a spitfire of a person, despite having macular degeneration
and late-stage congestive heart failure (CHF). Madeline had a very strong
spirit and was fiercely determined to maintain as much of her independence and control as possible. Her family contacted me because they
were at their wits' end with her, as Madeline was frequently going to the
emergency room to stabilize her condition. They hoped I could encourage her to accept palliative care. However, Madeline was a competent
adult and had lived on her own since her husband had died almost
thirty-five years ago.

I had a hunch from the beginning that trying to convince Madeline
would be an exercise in futility. And so I tried to connect to her in another
way. I told her how impressive it was that she could live for so long on
her own and that she must have a strong will and spirit. I pointed out
that if she wanted to stay out of the hospital, she would need to let others
help her. I reminded Madeline how many times she had been to the ER
and in the hospital, and how miserable she felt. I explained to her there
was a team of people who could help monitor her CHF and keep her
more comfortable.

Madeline latched onto the idea of staying out of the hospital. She
accepted palliative care and even enjoyed some of the team members'
visits. The team successfully kept her out of the hospital for quite some
time. Over time, however, her CHF became more difficult to control and
she was admitted into the hospital. This time, her condition was quite
serious. After four days in the hospital, her doctor and I agreed that
maybe her strong will and spirit were finally succumbing to her weak-
ened body and heart. The doctor informed her family that they might

want to prepare for her imminent death. With my support, Madeline was admitted to an inpatient hospice facility. Everyone was prepared for Madeline's death. In fact, her family donated her clothes and personal effects to a local charity.

Yet, to everyone's surprise, Madeline's strong spirit prevailed and her medical condition stabilized. In fact, when she learned that her children had given away her clothes, she ordered them to go find them and buy they back. Or better yet, take her to the thrift store. She was back to her old self. She had bounced back and won the heart of all the hospice staff and volunteers who worked with her. Within two months, Madeline had improved to the extent that she was released from hospice care. Upon her exit from hospice, she exclaimed, "I graduated!"

I include this story because it shows that not everyone goes to hospice to die. This is not to say that this will happen with your care recipient. Sometimes, as was the case with Madeline, hospice can actually improve the person's health. Madeline enjoyed another year of life before she died.

"I Can't Stand It Anymore" — A Daughter's Experience

Sharon came to me because she said she "couldn't stand to see her father suffer anymore." Her father had lung cancer that had metastasized to his brain. He was still living at home and had four hours a day of caregiver help. Sharon mentioned that her father was always a fighter and had told his doctor that he could "beat this beast." After two years, his cancer had metastasized to his brain. Yet he insisted on continuing treatment with more chemotherapy and radiation. Sharon stated that her father's oncologist was doing everything he could. In addition, Sharon believed her two siblings were in denial and struggling with the notion that their father was dying. They kept pushing their father to continue his various treatments. But Sharon was the one overseeing her father's care and the one seeing him suffer.

Sharon suspected her father was afraid of dying. She called me to help her determine what she could do to help her father and relieve some of her worry. When I met her father, I was shocked. He was weak, frail, and barely able to talk, slept most of the day, and was hardly eating or drinking. His last treatment had been two weeks earlier and the next one was scheduled in three days.

I called Sharon immediately and gently but firmly encouraged her to consider a hospice evaluation. I could hear the relief in her voice. She totally agreed and had been thinking about it for weeks. Fortunately, Sharon enlisted a nurse at her father's primary care doctor to convince the oncologist to order a hospice evaluation. Hospice came out and immediately started working with the family.

I received a call about a week later. Sharon's father had died. She praised the hospice team and said how wonderful and comforting it was to have them. And she said that the chaplain was able to help comfort her father around his fear of dying. In the last week of her father's life, Sharon was able to help him, and her, to "finish well." If you find yourself in a similar situation, ask if hospice may be of benefit to you.

"I Will Not Go Back to Rehab Again!" — Joe and His Son, Mark

Joe was ninety years old and had been living with CHF for the past fifteen years. For the third time in two months, he was hospitalized for his congestive heart failure. Joe was to be discharged in the next few days with an order for rehab, but Joe did not want to go. He had been there about a month earlier and told his son, Mark, that he was tired and just wanted to have some peace. He said he was ready to die. Mark met with the hospital discharge planner and told her that he didn't want rehab for his father. However, the discharge planner insisted that the doctor ordered rehab care and that was where her father would have to go. Mark felt completely overwhelmed and distraught. He called me. I talked to Mark and suggested I visit Joe in order to assess the situation. After meeting Joe, reading his chart, and talking with his nurses, it was very clear that a hospice evaluation was needed. However, it was not easy to get. I had to advocate and push for that order. Finally the doctor did write it. Joe not only qualified for hospice care but inpatient hospice care as well. Mark was so relieved. He knew in his heart that this was the best decision for his father. Mark called two weeks later to tell me that his father had died. He thanked me for helping get his father into hospice care.

I share this story because sometimes you have to advocate for what you want. And sometimes that means changing the course of direction, as was the case with Joe.

HEALTHY APPROACHES TO COPING WITH GRIEF AND LOSS

As most of you are aware, loss and grief often comes with major bumps in the road. And as Judith Viorst states, loss is indeed necessary.[3] Yet there are ways to cope that can ultimately lead to more ease and personal growth. As you journey through the last stages of caregiving, remember that the process is very personal and you will need to find coping strategies that feel comfortable to you.

Ways to Take Care of Yourself

Whether you have provided care for years or a short time, the end of your journey can be a mixed blessing, marked by a sense of relief and sadness. Being conscious of how you are feeling is critical to helping you maintain positive health and well-being. This stage of caregiving can offer a time of healing. For many of you, caring for someone at the end stages of a disease can provide an opportunity to reflect, quiet your mind, and connect to your heart. This time, more than ever, you need to be intentional about taking care of yourself. Focus on ways to replenish yourself, particularly paying attention to how your spirit feels. So what might be some positive ways to take care of yourself?

- Allow yourself to slow down and just be.
- Stay connected or reconnect to your spiritual resources.
- Make sure you are getting proper rest.
- Consider reaching out for professional help or joining a support group.
- Try physical outlets such as walking, swimming, or yoga, to name a few.
- Reach out to your friends and family. Tell them what you need. Perhaps they could cook some meals or be with your care recipient so you can go out for a movie or bite to eat.
- Find a creative outlet, such as drawing, journaling, or dancing.
- Make your own list of positive comforts.

Each caregiver will create his or her own path. My hope is you won't travel your path alone.

Religious and Spiritual Ways to Cope with Loss

> How do we find meaning amidst what appears to be a ruthless and meaningless process? Is it possible to find something redeeming while living with a heartbreaking illness?
> —Olivia Hoblitzelle, *Ten Thousand Joys & Ten Thousand Sorrows*, 2

At this time in your journey for those of you who have spiritual or religious orientation, your spiritual and religious beliefs can offer personal and community support. They can also offer ways for you to find meaning and even some peace.

When my mother was diagnosed with Alzheimer's disease, I made a conscious decision to find comfort and more ease in whatever ways I could. I was not a particularly religious person, nor was I a member of a synagogue—yet somehow I had a hunch that my Judaism might be helpful. I found a rabbi to talk to about end-of-life issues. After talking with the rabbi, I was incredibly surprised at the comfort and support I received from her wise counsel. She reminded me of the many Jewish practices, prayers, and rituals in which I could find refuge. She and I were also able to discuss my mother's funeral. And a week before my mother died, the rabbi came over and sat with me and we recited several prayers together. She also blessed my mother. I will always be grateful for that experience.

I share this because some of you may not be particularly religious or spiritual but may want to reconsider reconnecting and seeking out religious or spiritual comfort. For those of you who are, religion and spirituality can:

- Provide structure and rituals to guide you through difficult times
- Offer you a faith community that can support you
- Provide you with a place of refuge
- Challenge you to find ways to create meaning out of end of life
- Offer prayers that can sustain and comfort you
- Help you to focus inward and get in touch with your heart

Lastly, I encourage you to consider what other religions have to offer. I have found that some of the prayers, music, and rituals of other faiths provided additional comfort. They, along with my own religious rituals, sustained me through bereavement and mourning, and helped my healing.

Rituals of Remembering: Ways to Cope with Loss

> Rituals are a central part of life. . . . They connect us with our past, define our present life, and show us a path to our future as we pass on ceremonies, traditions, objects, symbols and ways of being with each other, handed down from previous generations.
> —Evan Imber-Black and Janine Roberts, *Rituals for Our Times*, 4

Every culture has rituals that guide its people through life's passages. Rituals connect us to our families, friends, and the larger community. Let's examine how rituals may help. Rituals can:

- Help us to feel that we belong
- Keep us connected to our families
- Provide support during passages
- Honor life's passages
- Celebrate our lives, individually and as a family or community
- Remind us of the transitions in life
- Provide anchors that can ground us
- Give us markers to pay tribute to our experiences

Before I present some ideas for creating rituals of remembering, I do want to mention that for some caregivers creating new rituals and or participating in past rituals can bring anguish and sadness. Some of you may be hesitant about creating rituals of remembering. Realize your feelings are normal because participating in old rituals you enjoyed with your care recipient can bring back happy memories, which can leave you feeling sad. However, as time passes you may gain some comfort in continuing or creating new rituals. My hope is that you will be able to either combine old rituals with new ones, or create new rituals that provide new ways to enjoy celebrations and holidays.

An innovative way to think about rituals is a concept that I call *rituals of remembering*. Rituals of remembering are ways to honor the memory of your care recipient that may be religious or nonreligious, familiar or new. Rituals can help you hold onto the memory of your care recipient. The following are some examples of rituals of remembering:

- Plant a tree or bush in your care recipient's honor. And perhaps on the anniversary of your care recipient's death, make a point to sit by the plant and reflect on your memories. You may also consider adding additional plants or flowers each year.
- Light a memorial candle. Jewish people often light a yahrzeit candle on the death of their loved one. Numerous non-Jewish caregivers have loved this idea.
- Celebrate a holiday your care recipient loved. For example, I always celebrate July 4 because it was my father's favorite holiday.
- Give yourself permission to talk to your care recipient when you need comforting or support. If this is not comfortable, consider trying doing so on her birthday, anniversary, or holiday time.
- Make a donation in your care recipient's memory on your care recipient's birthday or day he died.
- Consider becoming involved in an organization that represents your care recipient's prior illness, such as the Alzheimer's Association or Parkinson's Disease Association.
- Honor your care recipient at holidays or on special occasions, maybe even share heartwarming or funny stories.
- Wear an article of clothing that was special to your care recipient. For example, one client had her grandchildren wear a Braves baseball cap during their Passover Seder as a way of remembering their grandfather.
- Listen to your favorite song on the anniversary of your care recipient's death or birthday.

I leave you with a few final thoughts. Rituals of remembering can help validate the memory of your care recipient and honor your relationship. They can offer you renewed ways to keep the legacy of your care recipient's spirit alive. Hopefully this chapter helped you appreciate how loss can transform your life. End-of-life care can truly be one of the most sacred times in your life. And being able to "finish well" is a tribute to your courage, caring, and compassion.

NOTES

1. Terry D. Hargrave and William T. Anderson, *Finishing Well: Aging and Reparation in the Intergenerational Family* (New York: Routledge, 1992).

2. Elisabeth Kûbler-Ross, *On Death and Dying* (New York: Touchstone, 1969).

3. Judith Viorst, *Necessary Losses: The Loves, Illusions, Dependencies, and Impossible Expectations That All of Us Have to Give Up in Order to Grow* (New York: Fireside, 1998).

Appendix A

Key Information on Your Care Recipient

Throughout the book, I've talked about how to take care of yourself and your care recipient. In order to help the professionals who help you both, it is important to gather as much information as possible about your care recipient. I recommend that you collect the following key information:

- Medical Information
    1. List of each current medications, including names, doses, and prescribing physician
    2. Names and phone numbers of the primary care doctor
    3. Names and phone numbers of other health care providers and specialists
    4. Hospitalizations, including the dates and reasons
    5. Medical reports from other health professionals, such as physical therapy, speech therapy, or occupational therapy

- Cognitive History
    1. How the cognitive issues present themselves in your care recipient
    2. Neuropsychological reports (neuropsychological reports are a summation of the cognitive tests that were done on your care recipient).

- Psychological History
    1. History of depression, anxiety, paranoia, hallucinations, delusions

- Activities of Daily Living
    1. What personal care needs does your care recipient need help with, such as bathing, dressing, grooming, feeding, walking, and so forth

- Social History Information
    1. Place of birth
    2. Occupation
    3. Family history

4. Hobbies and interests
5. Religious and spiritual affiliations
6. Likes/dislikes
7. Important people and pets
8. Favorite past and current foods, activities

Appendix B

Caregiving Resources

HOW TO EVALUATE WEBSITES

The explosion of information on the Internet has its advantages and disadvantages. Finding information is easier and faster than ever before. But anyone can create a website, which makes finding reputable, quality information increasingly challenging. Before you believe what you read, hire a professional, purchase a service, or decide upon a health facility, it is critical to carefully evaluate the website. Here are some questions to help you do so.

- *Who sponsors the website?* The sponsor or hosting organization of the website should be apparent. Look for the name of the organization, agency, or party responsible for the site. Is it clear? Some websites, for example, exist for the sole purpose of selling a medication, product, or service. The sponsor may not always be disclosed. So look for information such as "about us." Reputable sites disclose who they are, who sponsors them (if applicable), and whether any organizations (government, nonprofit, business, commercial) have contributed funding, services, or material to the site.

- *What domain is the website?* Another clue to the sponsor is the domain name or the last three letters of the name. Certain domains are restricted, which means the site has to come from a particular organization, such as government (.gov), military (.mil), or educational institutions (.edu). Nonprofit organizations used to be designated by ".org" but this is no longer the case. Generally speaking, a website with a .com ending means it is a commercial enterprise. Sites with a .com ending may represent a specific individual, business, or company. They may also be a site sponsored by a company that uses the site to sell its goods and services. This does not mean that a commercial websites doesn't have valuable information; it means you need to understand its purpose and scrutinize the content. Federal and state government websites, which have a .gov ending, have an extensive review process and generally are more likely to have unbiased information. Their purpose is to provide information and there should not be any outside influence or conflict of interest on the site. Likewise, academic and educational institutions are committed to education and information and often strive to provide objective and unbiased information. Nonprofit professional organizations may provide useful information but sometimes push a particular agenda or cause. Commercial websites are supported through product sales, advertising, or sponsorship. As you see below, I have not recommended any commercial websites.

- *What is the purpose of the website?* The main purpose of the website should be evident. Is it to sell a product or service? Provide information? Share personal experiences? Look for a mission statement or a description of the organization. Does the information match your needs? Is the information unbiased? If you are looking to buy products or services, see if you can find an independent review or comparison. Companies exist to make a profit so they will naturally promote what they are selling. And as is the case with most things, there are good companies and not-so-good ones. So watch out for inflated claims, biased testimonials, or even false information.
- *Do they have contact information?* The site should provide contact information beyond an e-mail address or a form for you to submit. Look for a physical address and telephone number. If no physical address exists, be cautious, as the business may be virtual. This in and of itself may not be bad, but if you are looking for local services, you don't want to be talking to a call center halfway around the country.
- *What is the quality of the content?* Quality content has many different dimensions.

    1. *Are statements referenced or substantiated?* Where the information is coming from should be clear.
    2. *Is the information factual?* Make sure the information provided can be verified from an independent source. And are sources clearly identified?
    3. *How current is the information?* It should be reviewed and updated on a regular basis, especially medical information. Look for a notation of when the content was last reviewed or updated.
    4. *What is the expertise of the individual or organization?* If the website is a health professional, has the person explained his or her training, expertise, and licensed academic degrees? If the website is a business, can you independently validate their claims?
    5. *How is information created and reviewed?* This is particularly important for sites providing medical information. The site

should list the professional qualifications of the author, re-viewers, and/or editorial board.

6. *Does the site provide links to other credible sites?* Many sites will provide useful links to help you. But some sites will only list links if that organization has paid a fee. Is it clear how links are listed on the site?

- *Do they ask for personal information?* If a site is asking for personal information, look for a link that outlines what they do to protect your privacy. Do they clearly disclose what they do with your in-formation? For example, if they say they "share information with others," then your information isn't private. Make sure you are comfortable with their policy before you share your information.

- *Is information missing?* Sometimes you can tell more about a website by the information that is not there. For example, if a company talks about how many people they have helped but you can't find specif-ic information about their services and professionals, that may not be a good sign. If something doesn't feel right, it probably isn't. And if it's too good to be true, be skeptical.

ONLINE RESOURCES FOR CAREGIVERS

Below I have tried to provide some of the most widely used and re-spected national resources to help you with your caregiving journey. But since there are so many websites available and they change often, I list those I have determined are the most helpful national websites for care-givers.

Alzheimer's Association (www.alz.org)

The Alzheimer's Association is a national organization with a network of chapters in every state. It provides information, education, support, and referral. The Alzheimer's Association offers all kinds of services to caregivers and their care recipients.

Alzheimer's Store (www.alzstore.com)

The Alzheimer's store provides a variety of products and resources specifically geared to caregivers caring for a care recipient with dementia.

Alzheimer's Reading Room (www.alzheimersreadingroom.com)

The Alzheimer's Reading Room contains articles that offer a wide range of information for caregivers about Alzheimer's disease and related disorders.

American Association of Retired Persons (www.aarp.org;
(www.foundation.aarp.org/caregiving-resources.php)

AARP is a national organization offering information education, advocacy, and caregiving information for people over fifty. It also has a site related to the AARP Foundation that provides resources for caregivers.

American Health Care Association (www.ahcancal.org)

The American Health Care Association (AHCA) is the largest national association of long-term and postacute care providers. AHCA advocates for quality care and services for frail, elderly, and disabled individuals.

Family Caregiver Alliance (www.caregiving.org)

Family Caregiver Alliance offers information, education, and services for family caregivers, including the Family Care Navigator, a state-by-state list of services and assistance.

Leading Age (www.leadingage.org)

Leading Age is made up of not-for-profit organizations dedicated to helping older adults live safely and maintain as high a quality of life as possible. Leading Age advances policies and promotes practices in the long-term care industry.

Medicare (www.medicare.gov)

The official government site for Medicare provides information for those caring for a care recipient who qualifies for Medicare benefits.

National Academy of Elder Law Attorneys (www.naela.org)

The National Academy of Elder Law Attorneys is a professional association of attorneys who are dedicated to improving the quality of legal services provided to seniors and people with special needs.

National Adult Day Services Association (www.nadsa.org)

The National Adult Day Services Association is a professional membership organization comprised of adult day-services programs across the country. This organization provides information for caregivers about adult day care, advocacy, public policy, and research.

National Alliance for Caregiving (www.caregiving.org)

A coalition of national organizations focused on family caregiving issues, but the organization does not provide help to individuals.

National Family Caregivers Association (www.caregiveraction.org)

The National Family Caregivers Association is a nonprofit organization that provides information, resources, peer support, advocacy, and education to caregivers. They serve a broad spectrum of caregivers ranging from wounded soldiers and adults caring for aging parents to parents of children with special needs.

National Hospice and Palliative Care Organization (www.nhpco.org)

This is the largest national organization for American hospice programs. It offers general information on hospice and palliative care, and its website can point caregivers to local providers for these services.

National Institute on Aging (NIH) Alzheimer's Disease Education and Referral Center (www.nia.nih.gov/alzheimers)

The Alzheimer's Disease Education and Referral (ADEAR) Center is a service of the federal government's National Institute on Aging (NIA), one of the National Institutes of Health. The center provides accurate, up-to-date information about Alzheimer's disease and related disorders to patients and their families, caregivers, health care providers, and the public.

Strength for Caring (Johnson and Johnson) (www.strengthforcaring.com)

This website provides all kinds of resources, including support, caregiver tips, and caregiver online chat support with other caregivers. Strength for Caring is sponsored by Johnson and Johnson, who partners with other health care organizations.

The Administration on Aging (www.aoa.gov)

The Administration on Aging is a government agency in the newly formed Administration for Community Living. The website educates older people and their caregivers about the benefits and services that can help them.

The Joint Commission on Accreditation of Healthcare Organizations (www.jcaho.org)

A nonprofit organization that evaluates hospital care. This site can provide caregivers with information about how to handle concerns they might have while their care recipient is in the hospital.

The League of Experienced Family Caregivers (www4.uwm.edu/lefc)

The League of Experienced Family Caregivers (LEFC) is a registry of family members who care for their spouses, parents, elderly relatives, or wounded soldiers and who want to help other families by sharing information about their experiences as caregivers.

The National Consumer Voice for Quality Long-Term Care (www.theconsumervoice.org)

Advocates for consumer issues related to long-term care. The site provides a primary source of information and tools for consumers to help ensure quality of care for those in long-term care environments.

The NIH Senior Health (www.nihseniorhealth.gov)

NIH Senior Health contains information developed by the National Institute on Aging and the National Library of Medicine, both part of the federal government's National Institutes of Health. This website contains a wide range of information on many health topics for older adults, including Alzheimer's disease, arthritis, breast cancer, colorectal cancer, diabetes, taking medicines, and many more.

The Partnership for Prescription Assistance (www.pparx.org)

The Partnership for Prescription Assistance helps qualifying patients without prescription drug coverage get the medicines they need through the program that is right for them. Many will get their medications free or nearly free.

The Rosalynn Carter Institute for Caregivers (www.rosalynncarter.org)

The Rosalynn Carter Institute for Caregivers is an advocacy, education, research, and service unit of Georgia Southwestern State University. RCI provides caregivers with effective supports to promote caregiver health. RCI focuses on helping caregivers coping with chronic illness and disability across the lifespan.

Veterans Administration (www.va.gov; www.caregiver.va.gov)

The Department of Veteran Affairs website has information on VA programs, veterans' benefits, and facilities, as well as a specific site for caregivers of veterans.

Well Spouse Association (www.wellspouse.org)

The Well Spouse Association is an organization that provides support for well spouses caring for their ill spouses, whether due to illnesses of aging, accidents, or disease.

Bibliography

Albom, Mitch. *Tuesdays with Morrie*. New York: Random House, Inc., 1997.

Alzheimer's Association. "Alzheimer's Association." www.alz.org/.

A Tiny Treasure of African Proverbs. New York: Andrews McMeel, 1998.

Bartlett, John. *Bartlett's Familiar Quotations*, 17th ed. New York: Little Brown, 2002.

Bateson, Mary Catherine. *Composing a Further Life: The Age of Active Wisdom*. New York: Alfred A. Knopf, 2010.

Berman, Claire. *Caring for Yourself while Caring for Your Aging Parents*. New York: Henry Holt, 2006.

Boorstein, Sylvia. *It's Easier Than You Think: The Buddhist Way to Happiness*. New York: HarperCollins, 1997.

Boss, Pauline. *Loving Someone Who Has Dementia*. San Francisco: Jossey-Bass, 2011.

Brach, Tara. *Radical Acceptance: Embracing Your Life with the Heart of a Buddah*. New York: Bantam Books, 2003.

Burger, Sarah Greene, Virginia Fraser, Sara Hunt, and Barbara Frank. *Nursing Homes: Getting Good Care There*. Atascadero: Impact, 1996.

Centers for Disease Control and Prevention and the Kimberly-Clark Corporation. "Assuring Healthy Caregivers, a Public Health Approach to Translating Research into Practice: A Re-Aim Framework." 2008.

Cousins, Norman, and Rene Dubos. *Anatomy of an Illness as Perceived by the Patient: Reflections on Healing and Regeneration*. New York: W. W. Norton, 1979.

Dass, Ram. *Still Here: Embracing Aging, Changing, and Dying*. New York: Riverhead Books, 2000.

Fazio, Sam, Dorothy Saman, and Jane Stansall. *Rethinking Alzheimer's Care*. Baltimore: Professions Press, 1999.

Feng, Zhanlian, Brad Wright, and Vincent Mor. "Sharp Rise in Medicare Enrollees Being Held in Hospitals for Observation Raises Concerns about Causes and Consequences." *Health Affairs* 31, no. 6 (2012): 1251–59.

Friedman, Dayle A. *Jewish Visions for Aging: A Professional Guide for Fostering Wholeness*. Woodstock: Jewish Lights, 2008.

Gibran, Kahlil. *The Collected Works: Including Kahlil Gibran's Masterpiece, the Prophet Everyman's Library*. New York: Alfred A. Knopf, 2007.

Greenspan, Miriam. *Healing through the Dark Emotions: The Wisdom of Grief, Fear, and Despair*. Boston: Shambhala, 2004.

Hargrave, Terry D., and William T. Anderson. *Finishing Well: Aging and Reparation in the Intergenerational Family*. New York: Routledge, 1992.

Hoblitzelle, Olivia Ames. *Ten Thousand Joys & Ten Thousand Sorrows: A Couple's Journey through Alzheimer's*. New York: Penguin Group, 2008.

Hughes, Langston. *The Book of Negro Humor: Selected and Edited by Langston Hughes*. New York: Dodd, Mead, 1966.

Imber-Black, Evan, and Janine Roberts. *Rituals for Our Times: Celebrating, Healing, and Changing Our Lives and Our Relationships*. Lanham, Md.: Rowman & Littlefield, 1992.

Kay, Madeleine. *Living Serendipitously: Keeping the Wonder Alive*. Flat Rock: Chrysalis, 2003.

Keller, Hellen. *The Open Door*. New York: Doubleday, 1957.

Kornfield, Jack. *A Path with a Heart: A Guide through the Perils and Promises of Spiritual Life*. New York: Bantam Books, 1993.

Kûbler-Ross, Elisabeth. *On Death and Dying*. New York: Touchstone, 1969.

Kushner, Harold S. *Living a Life That Matters*. New York: Anchor Books, 2001.

Lade, Diane C. "Services Eager to Show Seniors the Way to a Home." *Sun Sentinel*, November 18, 2013.

Lerner, Harriet. *The Dance of Anger: A Woman's Guide to Changing the Patterns of Intimate Relationships*. New York: HarperCollins, 2005.

Levy, Naomi. *To Begin Again*. New York: Ballantine Books, 1998.

Luyster, Faith S., Patrick J. Strollo, Phyllis C. Zee, and James Walsh. "Sleep: A Health Imperative." *Sleep* 35, no. 6 (2012): 727–34.

Mace, Nancy L., and Peter V. Rabins. *The 36-Hour Day*. New York: Warner Books, 1999.

Machado, Antonio. "Traveller, There Is No Path."

Mayo Clinic. "Stress Relief from Laughter? Yes, No Joke." www.mayoclinic.com/health/stress-relief/SR00034/.

Medicare. "The Nursing Home Checklist." www.medicare.gov/nursing/checklist.pdf.

MetLife. "Adult Day Services." MetLife, 2010.

Miller, James E, and Susan C. Cutshall. *The Art of Being a Healing Presence*. Fort Wayne: Willowgreen, 2001.

The National Cancer Institute at the National Institutes of Health. "When Someone You Love Is Being Treated for Cancer." www.cancer.gov/cancertopics/coping/when-someone-you-love-is-treated.

Okun, Barbara, and Joseph Nowinski. *Saying Goodbye: How Families Can Find Renewal through Loss*. New York: Penguin Group, 2011.

Pipher, Mary. *Another Country: Navigating the Emotional Terrain of Our Elders*. New York: Berkley, 1999.

Reeves, Paula M. *Heart Sense: Unlocking Your Highest Purpose and Deepest Desires*. York Beach: Conari Press, 2003.

Remen, Rachel Naomi. *My Grandfather's Blessings: Stories of Strength, Refuge, and Belonging*. New York: Berkley, 2000.

Richards, Marty. *Caresharing: A Reciprocal Approach to Caregiving and Care Recieving in the Complexities of Aging, Illness or Disability*. Woodstock: SkyLight Paths, 2009.

Roosevelt, Eleanor. *You Learn by Living: Eleven Keys for a More Fulfilling Life*. Philadelphia: Westminster Press, 1960.

Roshi, Shunryu Suzuki. *Zen Mind, Beginner's Mind*. New York: Weatherhill, 1973.

Ruiz, Don Miguel. *The Four Agreements: A Practical Guide to Personal Freedom*. San Rafael: Amber-Allen, 2012.

Sandborn, Mark. *The Fred Factor*. New York: Doubleday, 2004.

Sarton, May. *As We Are Now: A Novel*. New York: W. W. Norton, 1973.

Seuss, Dr. *The Lorax*. New York: Random House, 1971.

Spiegel, David. "The Questionable Lure of Free Long-Term Care Placement Services." *Kaiser Health News* (July 11, 2013). www.kaiserhealthnews.org/Columns/2011/July/072811spiegel.aspx.

Strong, Maggie. *Mainstay*. Cambridge, Mass.: Bradford Books, 1997.

Tatelbaum, Judy. *The Courage to Grieve: Creative Living, Recovery and Growth through Grief*. New York: Lippincott and Crowell, 1980.

Ury, William. *The Power of a Positive No: Save the Deal, Save the Relationship, and Still Say No*. New York: Bantam Dell, 2007.

Viorst, Judith. *Necessary Losses: The Loves, Illusions, Dependencies, and Impossible Expectations That All of Us Have to Give Up in Order to Grow*. New York: Fireside, 1998.

Well Spouse Foundations. "Well Spouse Foundation." www.wellspouse.org.

Zona, Guy. *The Soul Would Have No Rainbow if the Eyes Had No Tears*. New York: Simon & Schuster, 1994.

Index

About the Author

Nancy L. Kriseman, LCSW, is a licensed clinical social worker who, for over thirty years, specializes in working with with elders and their families. Nancy is currently in private practice and also regularly consults with long-term care facilities. In addition, she conducts training and educational programs for families and caregivers for the Georgia Alzheimer's Association and a variety of other long-term care organizations and facilities. Nancy also brings her passion for older people into the classroom. She has been an adjunct faculty member at Mercer University and Kennesaw State University, where she has taught courses on "Aging and the Family" and "Death and Dying." Her previous book, *The Caring Spirit Approach to Eldercare: A Training Guide for Professionals and Families*, has won two national awards: Best Practices in Aging from the American Society on Aging and Hunter College and the other from the National Council on Aging, Mature Media award.

Ms. Kriseman holds a masters in social work and specialist in aging degree from the University of Michigan, 1982. She has her BA in psychology from the University of Florida, which she obtained in 1979.